Quick Reference
for
Health Care Providers

Prepared by:

Deborah E. Holmes, RN, CMA-C

Iowa Western Community College

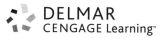

DELMAR
CENGAGE Learning™

Australia • Brazil • Japan • Korea • Mexico • Singapore • Spain • United Kingdom • United States

DELMAR
CENGAGE Learning™

Quick Reference for Health Care Providers
Deborah E. Holmes

Vice President, Health Care Business Unit: William Brottmiller

Editorial Director: Cathy L. Esperti

Acquisitions Editor: Marah Bellegarde

Editorial Assistant: Jennifer McGovern

Marketing Director: Jennifer McAvey

Marketing Coordinator: Kimberley Duffy

Senior Production Editor: James Zayicek

For product information and
technology assistance, contact us at **Cengage Learning Customer & Sales Support, 1-800-354-9706**
For permission to use material from this text or product, submit all requests online at **www.cengage.com/permissions**
Further permissions questions can be emailed to **permissionrequest@cengage.com**

Library of Congress Control Number: 2004049765

ISBN-13: 978-1-4018-5808-7

ISBN-10: 1-4018-5808-2

Delmar
Executive Woods
5 Maxwell Drive
Clifton Park, NY 12065
USA

Cengage Learning is a leading provider of customized learning solutions with office locations around the globe, including Singapore, the United Kingdom, Australia, Mexico, Brazil, and Japan. Locate your local office at **international.cengage.com/region**

Cengage Learning products are represented in Canada by Nelson Education, Ltd.

For your lifelong learning solutions, visit **delmar.cengage.com**

Visit our corporate website at **www.cengage.com**

Notice to the Reader

Publisher does not warrant or guarantee any of the products described herein or perform any independent analysis in connection with any of the product information contained herein. Publisher does not assume, and expressly disclaims, any obligation to obtain and include information other than that provided to it by the manufacturer. The reader is expressly warned to consider and adopt all safety precautions that might be indicated by the activities described herein and to avoid all potential hazards. By following the instructions contained herein, the reader willingly assumes all risks in connection with such instructions. The publisher makes no representations or warranties of any kind, including but not limited to, the warranties of fitness for particular purpose or merchantability, nor are any such representations implied with respect to the material set forth herein, and the publisher takes no responsibility with respect to such material. The publisher shall not be liable for any special, consequential, or exemplary damages resulting, in whole or part, from the readers' use of, or reliance upon, this material.

Printed in the United States of America
4 5 6 7 11 10

Contents

■ ■ ■

iii

Preface

■ ■ ■

Quick Reference for Health Care Providers is intended to be a reference guide that can be used by all health care students and practicing professionals. Students can use this reference to reinforce their classroom learning and memorizing. Practitioners will find this guide a quick way to verify stats and tips or a way to reinforce content that they may not use every day.

The first part of the book covers medical terminology. Section 1 covers medical terminology basics, including word parts and how to build medical terms. Section 2 lists commonly used word parts organized by English to word part and word part to English. This will allow the reader to find terms quickly and efficiently.

Section 3 lists common abbreviations and their meanings. Section 4 is a comprehensive conversions list of time, temperature, and measurement. Section 5 includes normal values for pulse, respiration, and temperature, and Section 6 contains tips for communicating with clients. Section 7 presents information on the three methods of dosage calculation, ways to calculate intravenous flow rates, and the seven rights of medication administration. Section 8 is a glossary, with definitions of common pathologies, and Section 9 contains a full-color collection of anatomical art that can be used for review.

This guide puts all this valuable information in one place. It can be used by students during their studies and right through their professional careers.

Medical Terminology Basics

■ ■ ■

WORD PARTS

The Three Types of Word Parts

Three types of word parts may be used to create medical terms.

- **Word roots**, also known as **combining forms**, contain the basic meaning of the term. They usually, *but not always*, indicate the involved body part.
- **Suffixes** usually, *but not always*, indicate the procedure, condition, disorder, or disease. A suffix always comes at the end of a word.
- **Prefixes** usually, *but not always*, indicate location, time, number, or status. A prefix always comes at the beginning of a word.

WORD ROOTS (COMBINING FORMS)

Word roots, also known as **combining forms**, act as the foundation of most medical terms. They usually, but not always, describe the part of the body that is involved.

Combining Vowels

To make the medical term easier to pronounce, a combining vowel may be needed between the word root and suffix. The rules for using combining vowels are explained in Table 1.1.

- The letter *O* is the most commonly used combining vowel.
- When a word root is shown with a backslash and a combining vowel, such as **cardi/o**, this is referred to as a **combining form** (**cardi/o** means heart).

SUFFIXES

A suffix is added to the end of a word root to complete the term. Suffixes usually, but not always, indicate the procedure, condition, disorder, or disease (Figure 1-1).

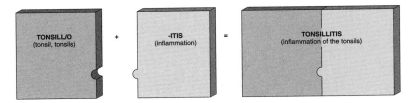

FIGURE 1-1 A word root (combining form) plus a suffix creates a new term.

- For example, **tonsill/o** means tonsils. A suffix is added to complete the term and tell what is happening to the tonsils.
- **Tonsillitis (ton-sih-LYE-tis)** is an inflammation of the tonsils (**tonsill** means tonsils and **itis** means inflammation).
- A **tonsillectomy (ton-sih-LECK-toh-mee)** is the surgical removal of the tonsils (**tonsill** means tonsils and **ectomy** means surgical removal).

PREFIXES

A prefix is added to the beginning of a word to change the meaning of that term. Prefixes usually, but not always, indicate location, time, or number. The term **natal (NAY-tal)** means pertaining to birth (**nat** means birth, and **al** means pertaining to). The following examples show how a prefix changes the meaning of this term.

- **Prenatal (pre-NAY-tal)** means the time and events before birth (**pre** means before, **nat** means birth, and **al** means pertaining to).
- **Perinatal (pehr-ih-NAY-tal)** refers to the time and events surrounding birth (**peri** means surrounding, **nat** means birth, and **al** means pertaining to). This is the time just before, during, and just after birth (Figure 1-2).
- **Postnatal (pohst-NAY-tal)** means the time and events after birth (**post** means after, **nat** means birth, and **al** means pertaining to).

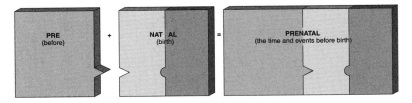

FIGURE 1-2 A prefix added to a word root (combining form) plus a suffix changes the meaning of the term.

DETERMINING MEANINGS BASED ON WORD PARTS

When you know the meaning of the word parts, it is often possible to figure out the definition of an unfamiliar medical term.

Taking Terms Apart

To determine a word's meaning by looking at the component pieces, you must first separate it into word parts.

- Most people like to start at the end of the word and work toward the beginning.
- Others like to start at the beginning of a word and work toward the end.
- Try it both ways. Then use the system that works best for you.

As an Example

Look at the term otorhinolaryngology. It is made up of three combining forms plus a suffix (Figure 1-3).

- The word root **ot/o** means ear. The combining vowel is used because ot/o is joining another word root.
- The word root **rhin/o** means nose. The combining vowel is used because rhin/o is joining another word root.
- The word root **laryng/o** means larynx and throat. The combining vowel *is not used* because laryng/o is joining a suffix that begins with a vowel.
- The suffix -ology means the study of.
- Together they form otorhinolaryngology (oh-toh-rye-noh-lar-in GOL-oh-jee), which is the study of the ears, nose, and throat (**oto** means ear, **rhino** means nose, **laryng** means throat, and **ology** means study of).
- Because this is such a long name, this specialty is frequently referred to as ENT (ears, nose, throat) or shortened to otolaryngology (oh-toh-lar-in-GOL-oh-jee).

SINGULAR AND PLURAL ENDINGS

Many medical terms have Greek or Latin origins. As a result of these different origins, there are unusual rules for changing a singular word into a plural form (Table 1.1). Additionally, English endings have been adopted for some commonly used terms.

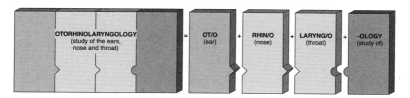

FIGURE 1-3 A medical term may be taken apart to determine its meaning.

TABLE 1.1 Guidelines to Unusual Plural Forms

Guideline	Singular	Plural
1. If the term ends in a, the plural is usually formed by adding an e.	bursa vertebra	bursae vertebrae
2. If the term ends in ex or ix, the plural is usually formed by changing the ex or ix to ices.	appendix index	appendices indices
3. If the term ends in is, the plural is usually formed by changing the is to es.	diagnosis metastasis	diagnoses metastases
4. If the term ends in itis, the plural is usually formed by changing the is to ides.	arthritis meningitis	arthritides meningitides
5. If the term ends in nx, the plural is usually formed by changing the x to ges.	phalanx meninx	phalanges meninges
6. If the term ends in on, the plural is usually formed by changing the on to a.	criterion ganglion	criteria ganglia
7. If the term ends in um, the plural usually is formed by changing the um to a.	diverticulum ovum	diverticula ova
8. If the term ends in us, the plural is usually formed by changing the us to i.	alveolus malleolus	alveoli malleoli

If you are in doubt as to how a plural is formed, look it up in a medical dictionary!

Medical Prefixes, Word Roots
(Combining Forms), and Suffixes

■ ▓ ▒

Pertaining to

-ac	pertaining to
-al	pertaining to
-ar	pertaining to
-ary	pertaining to
-eal	pertaining to
-ical	pertaining to
-ial	pertaining to
-ic	pertaining to
-ine	pertaining to
-ior	pertaining to
-ory	pertaining to
-ous	pertaining to
-tic	pertaining to

Abnormal Conditions

-ago	abnormal condition, disease
-esis	abnormal condition, disease
-ia	abnormal condition, disease
-iasis	abnormal condition, disease
-ion	condition
-ism	condition, state of
-osis	abnormal condition, disease

Noun Endings

-a	noun ending
-e	noun ending
-um	singular noun ending
-us	singular noun ending
-y	noun ending

MEDICAL WORD PART TO ENGLISH

A

a-, an-	no, not without, away from, negative
-a	noun ending
ab-	away from, negative, absent
abdomin/o	abdomen
-able	capable of, able to
abort/o	premature expulsion of a nonviable fetus
-ac	pertaining to
acanth/o	spiny, thorny
acetabul/o	acetabulum (hip socket)
-acious	characterized by
acous/o, acoust/o	hearing, sound
acr/o	extremities (hands and feet), top, extreme point
acromi/o	acromion, point of shoulder blade
actin/o	light
acu/o	sharp, severe, sudden
acuit/o, acut/o	sharp, sharpness
acust/o, -acusia, -acusis	hearing, sense of hearing
ad-	toward, to, in direction of
aden/o	gland
adenoid/o	adenoids
adhes/o	stick to, cling to
adip/o	fat
adnex/o	bound to
adren/o, adrenal/o	adrenal glands
aer/o	air, gas
aesthet/o	sensation, sense of perception
af-	toward, to
agglutin/o	clumping, stick together
aggress/o	attack, step forward
-ago	abnormal condition, disease
agor/a	marketplace
-agra	excessive pain, seizure, attack of severe pain
-aise	comfort, ease
-al	pertaining to
alb/i, alb/o, albin/o	white
albumin/o	albumin, protein
alg/e, algi/o, alg/o, algesi/o	relationship to pain
-algesia, -algesic	painful, pain sense
-algia	pain, painful condition
all/o, all-	other, different from normal, reversal
alveol/o	alveolus, air sac, small sac
ambi-	both sides, around or about, double

ambly/o	dull, dim
ambul/o, ambulat/o	walk
-amine	nitrogen compound
amni/o	amnion, fetal membrane
amph-	around, on both sides, doubly
amput/o, amputat/o	cut away, cut off a part of the body
amyl/o	starch
an-, ana-	up, apart, backward, excessive
an/o	anus, ring
-an	characteristic of, pertaining to
-ancy	state of
andr/o	related to the male
aneurysm/o	localized dilatation of the wall of a blood vessel
angi/o	blood or lymph vessels
angin/o	angina, choking, strangling
anis/o	unequal
ankyl/o	crooked, bent, stiff
anomal/o	irregularity
ante-	before, in front of
anter/o	before, front
anthrac/o	coal, coal dust
anti-	against
anxi/o, anxiet/o	uneasy, anxious, fearful
aort/o	aorta
ap-	toward, to
-apheresis	removal
aphth/o	ulcer
apic/o	apex
aplast/o	defective development, lack of development
ap-, apo-	separation, away from, opposed, detached
aponeur/o	aponeurosis (type of tendon)
apoplect/o	a stroke
append/o, appendic/o	appendix
aqu/i, aqu/o, aque/o	water
-ar	pertaining to
arachn/o	spider web, spider
arc/o	bow, arc, or arch
-arche	beginning
areat/o	occurring in patches or circumscribed areas
-aria	connected with
arter/o, arteri/o	artery
arteriol/o	arteriole
arthr/o	joint
articul/o	joint
-ary	pertaining to
as-	toward, to

-ase	enzyme
aspir/o, aspirat/o	to breathe in
asthen-, asthenia	weakness, lack of strength
asthmat/o	gasping, choking
astr/o	star, star-shaped
at-	toward, to
atel/o	incomplete, imperfect
ather/o	plaque, fatty substance
atop/o	strange, out of place
atres/i	without an opening
atri/o	atrium
attenuat/o	diluted, weakened
aud-, audi/o, audit/o	ear, hearing, the sense of hearing
aur/i, aur/o	ear, hearing
auscult/o	listen
aut/o	self
ax/o	axis, main stem
axill/o	armpit
azot/o	urea, nitrogen

B

bacill/o	rod-shaped bacterium (plural, bacteria)
bacteri/o	bacteria (singular, bacterium)
balan/o	glans penis
bar/o	pressure, weight
bartholin/o	Bartholin's gland
bas/o	base, opposite of acid
bi-, bis-	twice, double, two
bio-	life
bifid/o	split, divided into two parts
bil/i	bile, gall
bilirubin/o	bilirubin
bin-	two by two
-blast	embryonic, immature, formative element
blephar/o	eyelid
brachi/o	arm
brachy-	short
brady-	slow
brev/i, brev/o	short
bronch/i, bronchi/o, bronch/o	bronchial tube, bronchus
bronchiol/o	bronchiole, bronchiolus
brux/o	grind
bucc/o	cheek
burs/o	bursa, sac of fluid near joint
byssin/o	cotton dust

C

cadaver/o	dead body, corpse
calci-, calc/o	calcium
calcane/o	calcaneus, heel bone
calcul/o	stone, little stone
cali/o, calic/o	cup, calyx
call/i, callos/o	hard, hardened and thickened
calor/i	heat
canth/o	corner of the eye
capillar/o	capillary
capit/o	head
-capnia	carbon dioxide
capn/o	carbon dioxide, sooty or smoky appearance
capsul/o	little box
carb/o	carbon
carbuncl/o	carbuncle
carcin/o	cancerous
cardi/o, card/o	heart
cari/o	rottenness, decay
carot/o	stupor, sleep
carp/o	wrist bones
cartilag/o	cartilage, gristle
caruncul/o	bit of flesh
cat-, cata-, cath-	down, lower, under, downward
catabol/o	a breaking down
cathart/o	cleansing, purging
cathet/o	insert, send down
caud/o	lower part of body, tail
caus/o, caust/o	burning, burn
cauter/o, caut/o	heat, burn
cav/i, cav/o	hollow, cave
cec/o	cecum
-cele	hernia, tumor, swelling
celi/o, cel/o	abdomen, belly
cement/o	cementum, a rough stone
cent-	hundred
-centesis	surgical puncture to remove fluid
cephal/o, -ceps	head
cera-	wax
cerebell/o	cerebellum
cerebr/o	cerebrum, brain
cerumin/o	cerumen, earwax
cervic/o	neck, cervix (neck of uterus)
-chalasis, -chalasia	relaxation
cheil/o	lip
cheir/o	hand
chem/i, chem/o, chemic/o	drug, chemical

-chezia	defecation, elimination of waste
chir/o	hand
chlor/o	green
chlorhydr/o	hydrochloric acid
chol/e	bile, gall
cholangi/o	bile duct
cholecyst/o	gallbladder
choledoch/o	common bile duct
cholesterol/o	cholesterol
chondr/o	cartilage
chord/o	spinal cord, cord
chore/o	dance
chori/o, chorion/o	chorion, membrane
choroid/o	choroid layer of eye
chrom/o, chromat/o	color
chron/o	time
chym/o	to pour, juice
cib/o	meal
cicatric/o	scar
-cidal	pertaining to killing
-cide	causing death
cili/o	eyelashes, microscopic hairlike projections
cine-	relationship to movement
circ/i	ring or circle
circulat/o	circulate, go around in a circle
circum-	around, about
circumcis/o	cutting around
circumscrib/o	confined, limited in space
cirrh/o	orange-yellow, tawny
cis/o	cut
clasis, -clast	break down
claudicat/o	limping
claustr/o	barrier
clavicul/o, cleid/o	clavicle, collar bone
climacter/o	crisis, rung of a ladder
clitor/o	clitoris
clus/o	shut or close
-clysis	irrigation, washing
co-	together, with
coagul/o, coagulat/o	clotting, coagulation
coarct/o, coarctat/o	press together, narrow
cocc/i, cocc/o, -coccus	spherical bacteria
coccyg/o	coccyx, tailbone
cochle/o	spiral, snail, snail shell
coher/o, cohes/o	cling, stick together

coit/o	a coming together
col/o	colon, large intestine
coll/a	glue
colon/o	colon, large intestine
colp/o	vagina
column/o	pillar
com-	together, with
comat/o	deep sleep
comminut/o	break into pieces
communic/o	share, to make common
compatibil/o	sympathize with
con-	together, with
concav/o	hollow
concentr/o	condense, intensify, remove excess water
concept/o	become pregnant
conch/o	shell
concuss/o	shaken together, violently agitated
condyl/o	knuckle, knob
confus/o	confusion, disorder
coni/o	dust
conjunctiv/o	conjunctiva, joined together, connected
consci/o	aware, awareness
consolid/o	become firm or solid
constipat/o	pressed together, crowded together
constrict/o	draw tightly together
-constriction	narrowing
contact/o	touched, infected
contagi/o	infection, unclean, touching of something
contaminat/o	render unclean by contact, pollute
contra-	against, counter, opposite
contracept/o	prevention of conception
contus/o	bruise
convalesc/o	recover, become strong
convex/o	arched, vaulted
convolut/o	coiled, twisted
convuls/o	pull together
copi/o	plentiful
copulat/o	joining together, linking
cor/o	pupil
cord/o	cord, spinal cord
cordi/o	heart
core/o, cor/o	pupil
cori/o	skin, leather
corne/o	cornea
coron/o	coronary, crown
corp/u, corpor/o	body
corpuscul/o	little body
cort-	covering
cortic/o	cortex, outer region
cost/o	rib

cox/o	hip, hip joint
crani/o	skull
-crasia	a mixture of blending
creatin/o	creatine
crepit/o, crepitat/o	crackling, rattling
crin/o, -crine	secrete
cris/o, critic/o	turning point
-crit	to separate
cry/o	cold
crypt/o	hidden
cubit/o	elbow
cuboid/o	cubelike
culd/o	cul-de-sac, blind pouch
-cusis	hearing
cusp/i	point, pointed flap
cutane/o	skin
cyan/o	blue
cycl/o	ciliary body of eye, cycle
-cyesis	pregnancy
cyst-, -cyst	bladder, bag
cyst/o	urinary bladder, cyst, sac of fluid
cyt/o, -cyte	cell
-cytic	pertaining to a cell
-cytosis	condition of cells

D

dacry/o	tear, lacrimal duct (tear duct)
dacryocyst/o	lacrimal sac (tear sac)
dactyl/o	fingers, toes
de-	down, lack of, from, not, removal
debrid/e	open a wound
deca-, deci-	ten, tenth
decidu/o	shedding, falling off
decubit/o	lying down
defec/o, defecat/o	free from waste, clear
defer/o	carrying down or out
degenerat/o	gradual impairment, breakdown, diminished function
deglutit/o	swallow
dehisc/o	burst open, split
deliri/o	wandering in the mind
delt/o	Greek letter delta, triangular shape
dem/o	people, population
-dema	swelling (fluid)
demi-	half
dendr/o	branching, resembling a tree
dent/i, dent/o	tooth, teeth
depilat/o	hair removal
depress/o	press down lower, pressed or sunk down

derma-, dermat/o, derm/o	skin
desic/o	drying
-desis	surgical fixation of bone or joint, to bind, tie together
deteriorat/o	worsening or gradual impairment
dextr/o	right side
di-	twice, twofold, double
dia-	through, between, apart, complete
diaphor/o	sweat
diaphragmat/o	diaphragm, wall across
diastol/o	standing apart, expansion
diffus/o	pour out, spread apart
digit/o	finger or toe
dilat/o, dilatat/o	spread out, expand
-dilation	widening, stretching, expanding
dilut/o	dissolve, separate
diphther/o	membrane
dipl/o	double
dips/o, -dipsia	thirst
dis-	negative, apart, absence of
dislocat/o	displacement
dissect/o	cutting apart
disseminat/o	widely scattered
dist/o	far
distend/o, distent/o	stretch apart, expand
diur/o, diuret/o	tending to increase urine output
divert/i	turning aside
dors/i, dors/o	back of body
-dote	what is given
-drome	to run, running
-duct	opening
duct/o	to lead, carry
duoden/i, duoden/o	duodenum
dur/o	dura mater
-dynia	pain
dys-	bad, difficult, painful

E

-eal	pertaining to
ec-	out, outside
ecchym/o	pouring out of juice
ech/o	sound
eclamps/o, eclampt/o	flashing or shining forth
ectasia, -ectasis	stretching, dilation, enlargement
ecto-	out, outside

-ectomy	surgical removal, cutting out, excision
-ectopy	displacement
-edema	swelling
edem-, edemat/o	swelling, fluid, tumor
edentul/o	without teeth
effect/o	bring about a response, activate
effus/o	pouring out
ejaculat/o	throw or hurl out
electr/o	electricity, electric
eliminat/o	expel from the body
em-	in
-ema	condition
emaciat/o	wasted by disease
embol/o	something inserted or thrown in
embry/o	fertilized ovum, embryo
-emesis	vomiting
emet/o	vomit
-emia	blood, blood condition
emolli/o	make soft, soften
en-	in, within, into
encephal/o	brain
end-, endo-	in, within, inside
endocrin/o	secrete within
enter/o	small intestine
ento-	within
enzym/o	leaven
eosin/o	red, rosy
epi-	above, upon, on
epidemi/o	among the people, an epidemic
epididym/o	epididymis
epiglott/o	epiglottis
episi/o	vulva
epithel/i, epitheli/o	epithelium
equin/o	pertaining to a horse
-er	one who
erect/o	upright
erg/o, -ergy	work
erot/o	sexual love
eruct/o, eructat/o	belch forth
erupt/o	break out, burst forth
erythem/o, erythemat/o	flushed, redness
erythr/o	red
es-	out of, outside, away from
-esis	abnormal condition, disease
eso-	inward
esophag/o	esophagus
-esthesia, esthesi/o	sensation, feeling

esthet/o	feeling, nervous sensation, sense of perception
estr/o	female
ethm/o	sieve
eti/o	cause
eu-	good, normal, well, easy
-eurysm	widening
evacu/o, evacuat/o	empty out
ex-	out of, outside, away from
exacerbat/o	aggravate, irritate
exanthemat/o	rash
excis/o	cutting out
excori/o, excoriat/o	abrade or scratch
excret/o	separate, discharge
excruciat/o	intense pain, agony
exhal/o, exhalat/o	breathe out
exo-	out of, outside, away from
exocrin/o	secrete out of
expector/o	cough up
expir/o, expirat/o	breathe out
exstroph/o	turned or twisted out
extern/o	outside, outer
extra-	on the outside, beyond, outside
extrem/o, extremit/o	extremity, outermost
extrins/o	from the outside, contained outside
exud/o, exudat/o	to sweat out

F

faci/o	face, form
-facient	making, producing
fasci/o	fascia, fibrous band
fascicul/o	little bundle
fatal/o	pertaining to fate, death
fauc/i	narrow pass, throat
febr/i	fever
fec/i, fec/o	dregs, sediment, waste
femor/o	femur, thigh bone
fenestr/o	window
-ferent	carrying
-ferous	bearing, carrying, producing
fertil/o	fertile, fruitful, productive
fet/i, fet/o	fetus, unborn child
fibr/o	fiber
fibrill/o	muscular twitching
fibrin/o	fibrin, fibers, threads of a clot
fibros/o	fibrous connective tissue
fibul/o	fibula

-fic, fic/o	making, producing, forming
-fication	process of making
-fida	split
filtr/o, filtrat/o	filter, to strain through
fimbri/o	fringe
fiss/o, fissur/o	crack, split, cleft
fistul/o	tube or pipe
flamme/o	flame colored
flat/o	flatus, breaking wind, rectal gas
flex/o	bend
flu/o	flow
fluor/o	luminous, glowing
foc/o	focus, point
foll/i	bag, sac
follicul/o	follicle, small sac
foramin/o	opening, foramen
fore-	before, in front of
-form, form/o	resembling, in the shape of
fornic/o	arch, vault, brothel
foss/o	ditch, shallow depression
fove/o	pit
fract/o	break, broken
fren/o	device that limits movement
frigid/o	cold
front/o	forehead, brow
-fuge	to drive away
funct/o, function/o	perform, function
fund/o	bottom, base, ground
fung/i	fungus
furc/o	forking, branching
furuncul/o	furunculus, a boil, an infection
-fusion	pour

G

galact/o	milk
gamet/o	wife or husband, sperm or egg
gangli/o, ganglion/o	ganglion
gangren/o	eating sore, gangrene
gastr/o	stomach, belly
gastrocnemi/o	gastrocnemius, calf muscle
gemin/o	twin, double
gen-, gen/o, -gen	producing, forming
-gene	production, origin, formation
-genic, -genesis	creation, reproduction
genit/o	produced by, birth, reproductive organs
-genous	producing
ger/i, ger/o	old age

germin/o	bud, sprout, germ
geront/o	old age
gest/o, gestat/o	bear, carry young or offspring
gigant/o	giant, very large
gingiv/o	gingival tissue, gums
glauc/o	gray
glen/o	socket or pit
gli/o	neurologic tissue, supportive tissue of nervous system
globin/o, -globulin	protein
globul/o	little ball
glomerul/o	glomerulus
gloss/o	tongue
glott/i, glott/o	back of the tongue
gluc/o	glucose, sugar
glute/o	buttocks
glyc/o, glycos/o	glucose, sugar
glycer/o	sweet
glycogen/o	glycogen, animal starch
gnath/o	jaw
-gnosia	knowledge, to know
-gog, -gogue	make flow
goitr/o	goiter, enlargement of the thyroid gland
gon/e, gon/o	seed
gonad/o	gonad, sex glands
goni/o	angle
gracil/o	slender
grad/i	move, go, step, walk
-grade	go
-gram	resulting record
granul/o	granule(s)
-graph	instrument used for recording
-graphy	process of recording
gravid/o	pregnancy
-gravida	pregnant
gynce/o	woman, female
gyr/o	turning, folding

H

hal/o, halit/o	breath
halluc/o	great or large toe
hallucin/o	hallucination, to wander in the mind
hem/e	deep red iron-containing pigment
hem/o, hemat/o	blood, relating to the blood
hemangi/o	blood vessel
hemi-	half
hemoglobin/o	hemoglobin
hepat/o	liver
hered/o, heredit/o	inherited, inheritance

herni/o	hernia
heter/o	other, different
-hexia	habit
hiat/o	opening
hidr/o	sweat
hil/o	hilum, notch or opening from a body part
hirsut/o	hairy, rough
hist/o, histi/o	tissue
holo-	all
hom/o	same, like, alike
home/o	sameness, unchanging, constant
hormon/o	hormone
humer/o	humerus (upper arm bone)
hydr/o, hydra-	relating to water
hygien/o	healthful
hymen/o	hymen, a membrane
hyper-	excessive, increased
hypn/o	sleep
hypo-	deficient, decreased
hyster/o	uterus

I

-ia	abnormal condition, disease, plural of -ium
-iac	pertaining to
-ial	pertaining to
-ian	specialist
-iasis	abnormal condition, disease
iatr/o	physician, treatment
-iatrics	field of medicine, healing
-iatrist	specialist
-iatry	field of medicine
-ible	capable of, able to
-ic	pertaining to
-ical	pertaining to
ichthy/o	dry, scaly
-ician	specialist
icter/o	jaundice
idi/o	peculiar to the individual or organ, one, distinct
-iferous	bearing, carrying, producing
-ific	making, producing
-iform	shaped or formed like, resembling
-igo	attack, diseased condition
-ile	capable of
ile/o	ileum, small intestine
ili/o	ilium, hip bone
im-	not
immun/o	immune, protection, safe
impact/o	pushed against, wedged against, packed
impress/o	pressing into

impuls/o	pressure or pushing force, drive, urging on
in-	in, into, not, without
-in, -ine	a substance
-ine	pertaining to
incis/o	cutting into
incubat/o	incubation, hatching
indurat/o	hardened
infarct/o	filled in, stuffed
infect/o	infected, tainted
infer/o	below, beneath
infest/o	attack, assail, molest
inflammat/o	flame within, set on fire
infra-	below, beneath, inferior to
infundibul/o	funnel
ingest/o	carry or pour in
inguin/o	groin
inhal/o, inhalat/o	breathe in
inject/o	to force or throw in
innominat/o	unnamed, nameless
inocul/o	implant, introduce
insipid/o	tasteless
inspir/o, inspirat/o	breathe in
insul/o	island
insulin/o	insulin
intact/o	untouched, whole
inter-	between, among
intermitt/o	not continuous
intern/o	within, inner
interstiti/o	the space between things
intestin/o	intestine
intim/o	innermost
intoxic/o	put poison in
intra-	within, inside
intrins/o	contained within
intro-	within, into, inside
introit/o	entrance or passage
intussuscept/o	take up or receive within
involut/o	rolled up, curled inward
iod/o	iodine
-ion	action, process, state or condition
ion/o	ion, to wander
-ior	pertaining to
ipsi-	same
ir-	in
ir/i, ir/o, irid/o, irit/o	iris, colored part of eye
is/o	same, equal
isch/o	to hold back
ischi/o	ischium

-ism	condition, state of
iso-	equal
-ist	a person who practices, specialist
-itis	inflammation
-ium	structure, tissue
-ize	to make, to treat

J

jaund/o	yellow; jaundice
jejun/o	jejunum
jugul/o	throat
juxta-	beside, near, nearby

K

kal/i	potassium
kary/o	nucleus, nut
kel/o	growth, tumor
kera-	horn, hardness
kerat/o	horny, hard, cornea
ket/o, keton/o	ketones, acetones
kines/o, kinesi/o, -kinesia	movement
-kinesis	motion
klept/o	to steal
kraur/o	dry
kyph/o	bent, hump

L

labi/o	lip
labyrinth/o	maze, labyrinth, the inner ear
lacer/o, lacerat/o	torn, mangled
lacrim/o	tear, tear duct, lacrimal duct
lact/i, lact/o	milk
lactat/o	secrete milk
lamin/o	lamina
lapar/o	abdomen, abdominal wall
laps/o	slip, fall, slide
-lapse	to slide, fall, sag
laryng/o	larynx, throat
lat/i, lat/o	broad
later/o	side
lav/o, lavat/o	wash, bathe
lax/o, laxat/o	loosen, relax
leiomy/o	smooth (visceral) muscle
lemm/o	husk, peel, bark
-lemma	sheath, covering
lent/i	the lens of the eye
lenticul/o	shaped like a lens, pertaining to a lens
-lepsy	seizure

lept/o	thin, slender
-leptic	to seize, take hold of
letharg/o	drowsiness, oblivion
leuk/o	white
lev/o, levat/o	raise, lift up
libid/o, libidin/o	sexual drive, desire, passion
ligament/o	ligament
ligat/o	binding or tying off
lingu/o	tongue
lipid/o, lip/o	fat, lipid
-listhesis	slipping
lith/o, -lith	stone, calculus
-lithiasis	presence of stones
lob/i, lob/o	lobe, well-defined part of an organ
loc/o	place
loch/i	childbirth, confinement
-logy	study of
longev/o	long-lived, long life
lord/o	curve, swayback bent
lumb/o	lower back, loin
lumin/o	light
lun/o, lunat/o	moon
lunul/o	crescent
lup/i, lup/o	wolf
lute/o	yellow
lux/o	to slide
lymph/o	lymph, lymphatic tissue
lymphaden/o	lymph gland
lymphangi/o	lymph vessel
-lysis	breakdown, separation, setting free, destruction, loosening
-lyst	agent that causes lysis or loosening
-lytic	to reduce, destroy

M

macro-	large, abnormal size or length, long
macul/o	spot
magn/o	great, large
major/o	larger
mal-	bad, poor, evil
-malacia	abnormal softening
malign/o	bad, evil
malle/o	malleus, hammer
malleol/o	malleolus, little hammer
mamm/o	breast
man/i	madness, rage
man/i, man/o	hand
mandibul/o	mandible, lower jaw
-mania	obsessive preoccupation

manipul/o	use of hands
manubri/o	handle
masset/o	chew
mast/o	breast
mastic/o, masticat/o	chew
mastoid/o	mastoid process
matern/o	maternal, or a mother
matur/o	ripe
maxill/o	maxilla (upper jaw)
maxim/o	largest, greatest
meat/o	opening or passageway
medi/o	middle
mediastin/o	mediastinum, middle
medic/o	medicine, physician, healing
medicat/o	medication, healing
medull/o	medulla (inner section), middle, soft, marrow
mega-	large, great
-megaly	enlargement
mei/o	less, meiosis
melan/o	black, dark
mellit/o	honey, honeyed
membran/o	membrane, thin skin
men/o	menstruation, menses
mening/o, meningi/o	membranes, meninges
menisc/o	meniscus, crescent
mens/o	menstruate, menstruation, menses
menstru/o, menstruat/o	occurring monthly
ment/o	mind, chin
mes-, meso-	middle
mesenter/o	mesentery
mesi/o	middle, median plane
meta-	change, beyond, subsequent to, behind, after or next
metabol/o	change
metacarp/o	metacarpals, bones of the hand
metatars/o	bones of the foot between the tarsus and toes
-meter	measure, instrument used to measure
metr/i, metr/o, metri/o	uterus
-metrist	one who measures
-metry	to measure
mio-	smaller, less
micr/o, micro-	small
mictur/o, micturit/o	urinate
mid-	middle
midsagitt/o	from front to back, at the middle
milli-	one-thousandth

-mimetic	mimic, copy
mineral/o	mineral
minim/o	smallest, least
minor/o	smaller
-mission	to send
mitr/o	a miter having two points on top
mobil/o	capable of moving
mono-	one, single
monil/i	string of beads, genus of parasitic mold or fungi
morbid/o	disease, sickness
moribund/o	dying
morph/o	shape, form
mort/i, mort/o, mort/u	death, dead
mortal/i	pertaining to death, subject to death
-mortem	death
mot/o, motil/o	motion, movement
muc/o, mucos/o	mucus
multi-	many, much
muscul/o	muscle
mut/a	genetic change
mut/o	unable to speak, inarticulate
mutagen/o	causing genetic change
my/o	muscle
myc/e, myc/o	fungus
mydri/o	wide
mydrias/i	dilation of the pupil
myel/o	spinal cord, bone marrow
myocardi/o	myocardium, heart muscle
myom/o	muscle tumor
myos/o	muscle
myring/o	tympanic membrane, eardrum
myx/o, myxa-	relating to mucus

N

nar/i	nostril
narc/o	numbness, stupor
nas/i, nas/o	nose
nat/i	birth
natr/o	sodium
nause/o	nausea, seasickness
neo-	new, strange
necr/o	death
-necrosis	tissue death
nect/o	bind, tie, connect
nephr/o	kidney
nerv/o, neur/i, neur/o	nerve, nerve tissue
neutr/o	neither, neutral

nev/o	birthmark, mole
nid/o	next
niter-, nitro-	nitrogen
noct/i	night
nod/o	knot, swelling
nodul/o	little knot
nom/o	law, control
non-	no
nor-	chemical compound
norm/o	normal or usual
nuch/o	the nape
nucle/o	nucleus
nucleol/o	little nucleus, nucleolus
nulli-	none
numer/o	number, count
nutri/o, nutrit/o	nourishment, food, nourish, feed
nyct/o, nyctal/o	night

O

ob-	against
obes/o	obese, extremely fat
obliqu/o	slanted, sideways
oblongat/o	oblong, elongated
obstetr/i, obstetr/o	midwife, one who stands to receive
occipit/o	back of the skull, occiput
occlud/o, occlus/o	shut, close up
occult/o	hidden, concealed
ocul/o	eye
odont/o	tooth
-oid	like, resembling
-ole	little, small
olecran/o	elbow, olecranon
olfact/o	smell, sense of smell
olig/o	scanty, few
-ologist	specialist
-ology	the science or study of
-oma	tumor, neoplasm
om/o	shoulder
oment/o	omentum, fat
omphal/o	umbilical cord, the navel
onc/o	tumor
-one	hormone
onych/o	fingernail or toenail
o/o, oo/o	egg
oophor/o	ovary
-opaque	obscure
opac/o, opacit/o	shaded, dark, impenetrable to light

oper/o, operat/o	perform, operate, work
opercul/o	cover or lid
ophthalm/o	eye, vision
-opia	vision condition
-opsia, -opsis, -opsy	vision, view of
opt/i, opt/o, optic/o	eye, vision
-or	one who
or/o	mouth, oral cavity
orbit/o	orbit, bony cavity or socket
orch/o, orchid/o, orchi/o	testicles, testis, testes
-orexia	appetite
organ/o	organ
orgasm/o	swell, be excited
orth/o	straight, normal, correct
-ory	pertaining to
os-	mouth, bone
-ose	full of, pertaining to, sugar
-osis	abnormal condition, disease
-osmia	smell, odor
oss/e, oss/i, oste/o, ost/o	bone
ossicul/o	ossicle (small bone)
-ostomy	surgically creating an opening
-ostosis	condition of bone
ot/o	ear, hearing
-otia	ear condition
-otomy	cutting, surgical incision
-ous	pertaining to
ov/i, ov/o	egg, ovum
ovari/o	ovary
ovul/o	egg
-oxia	oxygen condition
ox/i, ox/o, ox/y	oxygen
oxid/o	containing oxygen
oxy-	swift, sharp, acid
-oxysm/o	sudden

P

pachy-	heavy, thick
palat/o	palate, roof of mouth
pall/o, pallid/o	pale, lacking or drained of color
palm/o	palm of the hand
palpat/o	touch, feel, stroke
palpebr/o	eyelid
palpit/o	throbbing, quivering
pan-	all, entire, every

pancreat/o	pancreas
papill/i, papill/o	nipple-like
papul/o	pimple
par-, para-	beside, near, beyond, abnormal, apart from opposite, along side of
par/o	to bear, bring forth, labor
-para	to give birth
paralys/o, paralyt/o	disable
parasit/o	parasite
parathyroid/o	parathyroid glands
pares/i	to disable
-paresis	partial or incomplete paralysis
paret/o	to disable
-pareunia	sexual intercourse
pariet/o	wall
parotid/o	parotid gland
-parous	having borne one or more children
paroxysm/o	sudden attack
-partum, parturit/o	childbirth, labor
patell/a, patell/o	patella, kneecap
path/o, -pathy	disease, suffering, feeling, emotion
paus/o	cessation, stopping
-pause	stopping
pector/o	chest
ped/o	child, foot
pedi/a	child
pedicul/o	louse (singular), lice (plural)
pelv/i, pelv/o	pelvic bone, pelvic cavity, hip
pen/i	penis
pend/o	to hang
-penia	deficiency, lack, too few
peps/i, -pepsia, pept/o	digest, digestion
per-	excessive, through
percept/o	become aware, perceive
percuss/o	strike, tap, beat
peri-	surrounding, around
perine/o	perineum
peristals/o, peristalt/o	constrict around
peritone/o	peritoneum
perme/o	to pass or go through
perone/o	fibula
perspir/o	perspiration
pertuss/i	intensive cough
petechi/o	skin spot
-pexy	surgical fixation
phac/o	lens of eye

phag/o	eat, swallow
-phage	a cell that destroys, eat, swallow
-phagia	eating, swallowing
phak/o	lens of eye
phalang/o	phalanges, finger and toe
phall/o	penis
pharmac/o, pharmaceut/o	drug
pharyng/o	throat, pharynx
phas/o	speech
-phasia	speak or speech
phe/o	dusky
pher/o	to bear or carry
-pheresis	removal
phil/o, -phila, -philia, -phil	attraction to, like, love
phleb/o	vein
phlegm/o	thick mucus
phob/o, -phobia	abnormal fear
phon/o, -phonia	sound, voice
phor/o	carry, bear, movement
-phoresis	carrying, transmission
-phoria	to bear, carry, feeling, mental state
phot/o	light
phren/o	diaphragm, mind
-phthisis	wasting away
-phylaxis	protection
physi/o, physic/o	nature
-physis	to grow
phyt/o, -phyte	plant
pigment/o	pigment, color
pil/i, pil/o	hair
pineal/o	pineal gland
pinn/i	external ear, auricle
pituit/o, pituitar/o	pituitary gland
plac/o	flat plate or patch
placent/o	placenta, round flat cake
plak/o, -plakia	plaque, plate, thin flat layer or scale
plan/o	flat
plant/i, plant/o	sole of foot
plas/i, plas/o	development, growth, formation
plas/o, -plasia	development, formation, growth
-plasm	formative material of cells
plasm/o	something molded or formed
plast/o	growth, development, mold
-plastic	pertaining to formation
-plasty	surgical repair
ple/o	more, many
-plegia	paralysis, stroke

-plegic	one affected with paralysis
pleur/o	pleura, side of the body
plex/o	plexus, network
plic/o	fold or ridge
-pnea	breathing
-pneic	pertaining to breathing
pne/o-	breath, breathing
pneum/o, pneumon/o	lung, air
pod/o	foot
-poiesis	formation, to make
-poietin	substance that forms
poikil/o	varied, irregular
pol/o	extreme
poli/o	gray matter of brain and spinal cord
pollic/o	thumb
poly-	many
polyp/o	polyp, small growth
pont/o	pons (a part of the brain), bridge
poplit/o	back of the knee
por/o	pore, small opening
-porosis	lessening in density, porous condition
port/i	gate, door
post-	after, behind
poster/o	behind, toward the back
potent/o	powerful
pract/i, practic/o	practice, pursue an occupation
prandi/o, -prandial	meal
-praxia	action, condition concerning the performance of movements
-praxis	act, activity, practice use
pre-	before, in front of
precoc/i	early, premature
pregn/o	pregnant, full of
prematur/o	too early, untimely
preputi/o	foreskin, prepuce
presby/o	old age
priap/o	penis
primi-	first
pro-	before, in behalf of
process/o	going forth
procreat/o	reproduce
proct/o	anus and rectum
prodrom/o	running ahead, precursor
product/o	lead forward, yield, produce
prolaps/o	fall downward, slide forward
prolifer/o	reproduce, bear offspring
pron/o, pronat/o	bent forward
pros-	before

prostat/o	prostate gland
prosth/o, prosthet/o	addition, appendage
prot/o, prote/o	first
protein/o	protein
proxim/o	near
prurit/o	itching
pseud/o	false
psych/o	mind
-ptosis	droop, sag, prolapse, fall
-ptyal/o	saliva
-ptysis	spitting
pub/o	pubis, part of hip bone
pubert/o	ripe age, adult
pudend/o	pudendum
puerper/i	childbearing, labor
pulm/o, pulmon/o	lung
puls/o	beat, beating, striking
punct/o	sting, prick, puncture
pupill/o	pupil
pur/o	pus
purpur/o	purple
purul/o	pus-filled
pustul/o	infected pimple
py/o	pus
pyel/o	renal pelvis, bowl of kidney
pylor/o	pylorus, pyloric sphincter
pyr/o, pyret/o, pyrex/o	fever, fire
pyramid/o	pyramid shaped

Q

quadr/i, quadr/o	four

R

rabi/o	madness, rage
rachi/o	spinal column, vertebrae
radi/o	radiation, x-rays, radius (lateral lower arm bone)
radiat/o	giving off rays or radiant energy
radicul/o	nerve root
raph/o	seam, suture
re-	back, again
rect/o	rectum, straight
recuperat/o	recover, regain health
reduct/o	bring back together
refract/o	bend back, turn aside
regurgit/o	flood or gush back
remiss/o	give up, let go, relax

ren/o	kidney
resuscit/o	revive
retent/o	hold back
reticul/o	network
retin/o	retina, net
retro-	behind, backward, back of
retract/o	draw back or in
rhabdomy/o	striated muscle
rheum/o, rheumat/o	watery flow, subject to flow
rhin/o	nose
rhiz/o	root
rhonc/o	snore, snoring
rhythm/o	rhythm
rhytid/o	wrinkle
rigid/o	stiff
ris/o	laugh
roentgen/o	x-ray
rotat/o	rotate, revolve
-rrhage, -rrhagia	bleeding, abnormal excessive fluid discharge
-rrhaphy	to suture
-rrhea	abnormal flow, discharge
-rrhexis	rupture
rube-	red
rug/o	wrinkle, fold

S

sacc/i, sacc/o	sac
facchar/o	sugar
sacr/o	sacrum
saliv/o	saliva
salping/o	uterine (fallopian) tube, auditory (eustachian) tube
-salpinx	uterine (fallopian) tube
san/o	sound, healthy, sane
sangu/i, sanguin/o	blood
sanit/o	soundness, health
sapr/o	decaying, rotten
sarc/o	flesh, connective tissue
scapul/o	scapula, shoulder blade
schiz/o	division, split
scintill/o	spark
scirrh/o	hard
scler/o	sclera, white of eye, hard
-sclerosis	abnormal hardening
scoli/o	curved, bent
-scope	instrument for visual examination
-scopy	visual examination
scot/o	darkness

scrib/o, script/o	write
scrot/o	bag or pouch
seb/o	sebum
secret/o	produce, separate out
sect/o, secti/o	cut, cutting
segment/o	pieces
sell/o	saddle
semi-	half
semin/i	semen, seed, sperm
sen/i	old
senesc/o	grow old
senil/o	old age
sens/i	feeling, sensation
sensitiv/o	sensitive to, affected by
seps/o	infection
sept/o	infection, partition
ser/o	serum
seros/o	serous
sial/o	saliva
sialaden/o	salivary gland
sider/o	iron
sigmoid/o	sigmoid colon
silic/o	glass
sin/o, sin/u	hollow, sinus
sinistr/o	left, left side
sinus/o	sinus
-sis	abnormal condition, disease
sit/u	place
skelet/o	skeleton
soci/o	companion, fellow being
-sol	solution
solut/o, solv/o	loosened, dissolved
soma-, somat/o	body
somn/i, somn/o	sleep
son/o	sound
sopor/o	sleep
spad/o	draw off, draw
-spasm, spasmod/o	sudden involuntary contraction, tightening or cramping
spec/i	look at, a kind or sort
specul/o	mirror
sperm/o, spermat/	sperm, spermatozoa, seed
sphen/o	sphenoid bone, wedge
spher/o	round, sphere, ball
sphincter/o	tight band
sphygm/o	pulse
spin/o	spine, backbone
spir/o	to breathe
spirill/o	little coil

spirochet/o	coiled microorganism
splen/o	spleen
spondyl/o	vertebrae, vertebral column, back bone
spontane/o	unexplained, of one's own accord
spor/o	seed, spore
sput/o	sputum, spit
squam/o	scale
-stalsis	contraction, constriction
staped/o, stapedi/o	stapes (middle ear bone)
staphyl/o	clusters, bunch of grapes
-stasis, -static	control, maintenance of a constant level
steat/o	fat, lipid, sebum
sten/o	narrowing, contracted
-stenosis	abnormal narrowing
ster/o	solid structure
stere/o	solid, three-dimensional
steril/i	sterile
stern/o	sternum, the breastbone
stert/o	snore, snoring
steth/o	chest
-sthenia	strength
stigmat/o	point, spot
stimul/o	goad, prick, incite
stomat/o	mouth
-stomosis, -stomy	furnish with a mouth or outlet, new opening
strab/i	squint, squint-eyed
strat/i	layer
strept/o	twisted chain
striat/o	stripe, furrow, groove
stric-	narrowing
strict/o	draw tightly together, bind or tie
strid/o	harsh sound
styl/o	pen, pointed instrument
sub-	under, less, below
subluxat/o	partial dislocation
sucr/o	sugar
sudor/i	sweat
suffoc/o, suffocat/o	choke, strangle
sulc/o	furrow, groove
super-, super/o	above, excessive, higher than
superflu/o	overflowing, excessive
supin/o	lying on the back
supinat/o	bend backward, place on the back
suppress/o	press down
suppur/o, suppurat/o	to form pus

supra-	above, upper, excessive
sutur/o	stitch, seam
sym-	with, together, joined together
symptomat/o	falling together, symptom
syn-	together, with, union, association
synaps/o, synapt/o	point of contact
syncop/o	to cut short, cut off
-syndesis	surgical fixation of vertebrae
syndesm/o	ligament
syndrom/o	running together
synovi/o, synov/o	synovial membrane, synovial fluid
syphil/i, syphil/o	syphilis
syring/o	tube
system/o, systemat/o	body system
systol/o	contraction

T

tachy-	fast, rapid
tact/i	touch
tars/o	tarsus (ankle bone), instep, edge of the eyelid
tax/o	coordination, order
techn/o, techni/o	skill
tele/o	distant, far
tempor/o	temporal bone, temple
ten/o, tend/o	tendon, stretch out, extend, strain
tenac/i	holding fast, sticky
tendin/o	tendon
tens/o	stretch out, extend, strain
terat/o	malformed fetus, monster
termin/o	end, limit
test/i, test/o, testicul/o	testis, testicle
tetan/o	rigid, tense
tetra-	four
thalam/o	thalamus, inner room
thalass/o	sea
thanas/o, thanat/o	death
the/o	put, place
thec/o	sheath
thel/o	nipple
therap/o, therapeut/o	treatment
therm/o	heat
thio-	sulfur
thora/o, thorac/o	chest

-thorax	chest, pleural cavity
thromb/o	clot
thym/o	thymus gland, soul
-thymia	mind
-thymic	pertaining to the mind
thyr/o, thyroid/o	thyroid gland
tibi/o	tibia (shin bone)
-tic	pertaining to
tine/o	gnawing worm, ringworm
tinnit/o	ringing, buzzing, tinkling
-tion	process, state or quality of
toc/o, -tocia, -tocin	labor, birth
tom/o	cut, section, slice
-tome	instrument to cut
-tomy	process of cutting
ton/o	tension, tone, stretching
tone/o	to stretch
tonsill/o	tonsil, throat
top/o	place, position, location
tors/o	twist, rotate
tort/i	twisted
tox/o, toxic/o	poison, poisonous
trache/i, trache/o	trachea, windpipe
trachel-	neck
tranquil/o	quiet, calm, tranquil
trans-	across, through
transfus/o	pour across, transfer
transit/o	changing
transvers/o	across, crosswise
traumat/o	injury
trem/o	shaking, trembling
tremul/o	fine tremor or shaking
-tresia	opening
tri-	three
trich/o	hair
trigon/o	trigone
-tripsy	to crush
-trite	instrument for crushing
trop/o, -tropia	turn, change
troph/o, -trophy	development, nourishment
-tropic	turning
-tropin	stimulate, act on
tub/i, tub/o	tube, pipe
tubercul/o	little knot, swelling
tunic/o	covering, cloak, sheath
turbinat/o	coiled, spiral shaped
tuss/i	cough
tympan/o	tympanic membrane, eardrum
-type	classification, picture

U

-ula	small, little
-ule	small one
ulcer/o	sore, ulcer
uln/o	ulna (medial lower arm bone)
ultra-	beyond, excess
-um	singular noun ending
umbilic/o	navel
un-	not
ungu/o	nail
uni-	one
ur/o	urine, urinary tract
-uresis	urination
ureter/o	ureter
urethr/o	urethra
-uria	urination, urine
urin/o	urine or urinary organs
urtic/o	nettle, rash, hives
-us	thing, singular noun ending
uter/i, uter/o	uterus
uve/o	iris, choroid, ciliary body, uveal tract
uvul/o	uvula, little grape

V

vaccin/i, vaccin/o	vaccine
vag/o	vagus nerve, wandering
vagin/o	vagina
valg/o	bent or twisted outward
valv/o, valvul/o	valve
var/o	bent or twisted inward
varic/o	varicose veins, swollen or dilated vein
vas/o	vas deferens, vessel
vascul/o	blood vessel, little vessel
vast/o	vast, great, extensive
vect/o	carry, convey
ven/o	vein
vener/o	sexual intercourse
venter-	abdomen
ventilat/o	expose to air, fan
ventr/o	in front, belly side of body
ventricul/o	ventricle of brain or heart, small chamber
venul/o	venule, small vein
verm/i	worm
verruc/o	wart
-verse, -version	to turn
vers/o, vert/o	turn
vertebr/o	vertebra, backbone
vertig/o, vertigin/o	whirling round

vesic/o	urinary bladder
vesicul/o	seminal vesicle, blister, little bladder
vestibul/o	entrance, vestibule
vir/o	poison, virus
viril/o	masculine, manly
vis/o	seeing, sight
visc/o	sticky
viscer/o	viscera, internal organ
viscos/o	sticky
vit/a, vit/o	life
vitre/o	glassy, made of glass
viv/l	life
voc/i	voice
vol/o	palm or sole
volv/o	roll, turn
vulgar/i	common
vulv/o	vulva, covering

X

xanth/o	yellow
xen/o	strange, foreign
xer/o	dry
xiph/i, xiph/o	sword

Y

-y	noun ending

Z

zo/o	animal life
zygomat/o	cheek bone, yoke
zygot/o	joined together

ENGLISH TO MEDICAL WORD PART

A

abdomen	abdomin/o
abdomen	venter-
abdomen, abdominal wall	lapar/o
abdomen, belly	celi/o, cel/o
abnormal condition, disease, plural of -ium	-ia
abnormal condition, disease	-ago
abnormal condition, disease	-esis
abnormal condition, disease	-iasis
abnormal condition, disease	-osis
abnormal condition, disease	-sis
abnormal fear	phob/o, -phobia
abnormal flow, discharge	-rrhea
abnormal hardening	-sclerosis
abnormal narrowing	-stenosis
abnormal softening	-malacia
above, excessive, higher than	super-, super/o
above, upon, on	epi-
above, upper, excessive	supra-
abrade or scratch	excori/o, excoriat/o
acetabulum (hip socket)	acetabul/o
acromion, point of shoulder blade	acromi/o
across, crosswise	transvers/o
across, through	trans-
act, activity, practice use	-praxis
action, condition concerning the performance of movements	-praxia
action, process, state or condition	-ion
addition, appendage	prosth/o, prosthet/o
adenoids	adenoid/o
adrenal glands	adren/o, adrenal/o
after, behind	post-
against	anti-
against	ob-
against, counter, opposite	contra-
agent that causes lysis or loosening	-lyst
aggravate, irritate	exacerbat/o
air, gas	aer/o
albumin, protein	albumin/o
all, entire, every	pan-
all	holo-
alveolus, air sac, small sac	alveol/o
amnion, fetal membrane	amni/o
among the people, an epidemic	epidemi/o
angina, choking, strangling	angin/o
angle	goni/o

animal life	zo/o
anus and rectum	proct/o
anus, ring	an/o
aorta	aort/o
apex	apic/o
aponeurosis (type of tendon)	aponeur/o
appendix	append/o, appendic/o
appetite	-orexia
arch, vault, brothel	fornic/o
arched, vaulted	convex/o
arm	brachi/o
armpit	axill/o
around, about	circum-
around, on both sides, doubly	amph-
arteriole	arteriol/o
artery	arter/o, arteri/o
atrium	atri/o
attack, assail, molest	infest/o
attack, diseased condition	-igo
attack, step forward	aggress/o
attraction to, like, love	phil/o, -phila, -philia, -phil
aware, awareness	consci/o
away from, negative, absent	ab-
axis, main stem	ax/o

B

back, again	re-
back of body	dors/i, dors/o
back of the knee	poplit/o
back of the skull, occiput	occipit/o
back of the tongue	glott/i, glott/o
bacteria (singular, bacterium)	bacteri/o
bad, difficult, painful	dys-
bad, evil	malign/o
bad, poor, evil	mal-
bag or pouch	scrot/o
bag, sac	foll/i
barrier	claustr/o
Bartholin's gland	bartholin/o
base, opposite of acid	bas/o
bear, bring forth, labor	par/o
bear, carry, feeling, mental state	-phoria
bear or carry	pher/o
bear, carry young or offspring	gest/o, gestat/o
bearing, carrying, producing	-ferous
bearing, carrying, producing	-iferous
beat, beating, striking	puls/o

become aware, perceive	percept/o
become firm or solid	consolid/o
become pregnant	concept/o
before	pros-
before, front	anter/o
before, in behalf of	pro-
before, in front of	ante-
before, in front of	fore-
before, in front of	pre-
beginning	-arche
behind, backward, back of	retro-
behind, toward the back	poster/o
belch forth	eruct/o, eructat/o
below, beneath	infer/o
below, beneath, inferior to	infra-
bend	flex/o
bend back, turn aside	refract/o
bend backward, place on the back	supinat/o
bent forward	pron/o, pronat/o
bent, hump	kyph/o
bent or twisted inward	var/o
bent or twisted outward	valg/o
beside, near, beyond, abnormal, apart from opposite, along side of	par-, para-
beside, near, nearby	juxta-
between, among	inter-
beyond, excess	ultra-
bile duct	cholangi/o
bile, gall	bil/i
bile, gall	chol/e
bilirubin	bilirubin/o
bind, tie, connect	nect/o
binding or tying off	ligat/o
birth	nat/i
birthmark, mole	nev/o
bit of flesh	caruncul/o
black, dark	melan/o
bladder, bag	cyst-, -cyst
bleeding, abnormal excessive fluid discharge	-rrhage, -rrhagia
blood	sangu/i, sanguin/o
blood or lymph vessels	angi/o
blood vessel, little vessel	vascul/o
blood vessel	hemangi/o
blood, blood condition	-emia
blood, relating to the blood	hem/o, hemat/o
blue	cyan/o
body	corp/u, corpor/o
body	soma-, somat/o
body system	system/o, systemat/o

bone	oss/e, oss/i, oste/o, ost/o
bones of the foot between the tarsus and toes	metatars/o
both sides, around or about, double	ambi-
bottom, base, ground	fund/o
bound to	adnex/o
bow, arc, or arch	arc/o
brain	encephal/o
branching, resembling a tree	dendr/o
break, broken	fract/o
break down	clasis, -clast
break into pieces	comminut/o
break out, burst forth	erupt/o
breakdown, separation, setting free, destruction, loosening	-lysis
breaking down	catabol/o
breast	mamm/o
breast	mast/o
breath	hal/o, halit/o
breath, breathing	pne/o-
breathe	spir/o
breathe in	aspir/o, aspirat/o
breathe in	inhal/o, inhalat/o
breathe in	inspir/o, inspirat/o
breathe out	exhal/o, exhalat/o
breathe out	expir/o, expirat/o
breathing	-pnea
bring about a response, activate	effect/o
bring back together	reduct/o
broad	lat/i, lat/o
bronchial tube, bronchus	bronch/i, bronchi/o, bronch/o
bronchiole, bronchiolus	bronchiol/o
bruise	contus/o
bud, sprout, germ	germin/o
burning, burn	caus/o, caust/o
bursa, sac of fluid near joint	burs/o
burst open, split	dehisc/o
buttocks	glute/o

C

calcaneus, heel bone	calcane/o
calcium	calci-, calc/o
cancerous	carcin/o
capable of moving	mobil/o
capable of, able to	-able
capable of, able to	-ible
capable of	-ile

capillary	capillar/o
carbon	carb/o
carbon dioxide	-capnia
carbon dioxide, sooty or smoky appearance	capn/o
carbuncle	carbuncl/o
carry, bear, movement	phor/o
carry, convey	vect/o
carry or pour in	ingest/o
carrying	-ferent
carrying down or out	defer/o
carrying, transmission	-phoresis
cartilage	chondr/o
cartilage, gristle	cartilag/o
cause	eti/o
causing death	-cide
causing genetic change	mutagen/o
cecum	cec/o
cell	cyt/o, -cyte
cell that destroys, eat, swallow	-phage
cementum, a rough stone	cement/o
cerebellum	cerebell/o
cerebrum, brain	cerebr/o
cerumen, earwax	cerumin/o
cessation, stopping	paus/o
change	metabol/o
change, beyond, subsequent to, behind, after or next	meta-
changing	transit/o
characteristic of, pertaining to	-an
characterized by	-acious
cheek	bucc/o
cheek bone, yoke	zygomat/o
chemical compound	nor-
chest	pector/o
chest	steth/o
chest	thora/o, thorac/o
chest, pleural cavity	-thorax
chew	masset/o
chew	mastic/o, masticat/o
child	pedi/a
child, foot	ped/o
childbearing, labor	puerper/i
childbirth, confinement	loch/i
childbirth, labor	-partum, parturit/o
choke, strangle	suffoc/o, suffocat/o
cholesterol	cholesterol/o
chorion, membrane	chori/o, chorion/o
choroid layer of eye	choroid/o
ciliary body of eye, cycle	cycl/o
circulate, go around in a circle	circulat/o

classification, picture	-type
clavicle, collar bone	clavicul/o, cleid/o
cleansing, purging	cathart/o
cling, stick together	coher/o, cohes/o
clitoris	clitor/o
clot	thromb/o
clotting, coagulation	coagul/o, coagulat/o
clumping, stick together	agglutin/o
clusters, bunch of grapes	staphyl/o
coal, coal dust	anthrac/o
coccyx, tailbone	coccyg/o
coiled microorganism	spirochet/o
coiled, spiral shaped	turbinat/o
coiled, twisted	convolut/o
cold	cry/o
cold	frigid/o
colon, large intestine	col/o
colon, large intestine	colon/o
color	chrom/o, chromat/o
comfort, ease	-aise
coming together	coit/o
common	vulgar/i
common bile duct	choledoch/o
companion, fellow being	soci/o
condense, intensify, remove excess water	concentr/o
condition	-ema
condition of bone	-ostosis
condition of cells	-cytosis
condition, state of	-ism
confined, limited in space	circumscrib/o
confusion, disorder	confus/o
conjunctiva, joined together, connected	conjunctiv/o
connected with	-aria
constrict around	peristals/o, peristalt/o
contained within	intrins/o
containing oxygen	oxid/o
contraction	systol/o
contraction, constriction	-stalsis
control, maintenance of a constant level	-stasis, -static
coordination, order	tax/o
cord, spinal cord	cord/o
cornea	corne/o
corner of the eye	canth/o
coronary, crown	coron/o
cortex, outer region	cortic/o
cotton dust	byssin/o
cough up	expector/o

cough	tuss/i
cover or lid	opercul/o
covering	cort-
covering, cloak, sheath	tunic/o
crack, split, cleft	fiss/o, fissur/o
crackling, rattling	crepit/o, crepitat/o
creatine	creatin/o
creation, reproduction	-genic, -genesis
crescent	lunul/o
crisis, rung of a ladder	climacter/o
crooked, bent, stiff	ankyl/o
crush	-tripsy
cubelike	cuboid/o
cul-de-sac, blind pouch	culd/o
cup, calyx	cali/o, calic/o
curve, swayback bent	lord/o
curved, bent	scoli/o
cut	cis/o
cut away, cut off a part of the body	amput/o, amputat/o
cut, cutting	sect/o, secti/o
cut, section, slice	tom/o
cut short, cut off	syncop/o
cutting apart	dissect/o
cutting around	circumcis/o
cutting into	incis/o
cutting out	excis/o
cutting, surgical incision	-otomy

D

dance	chore/o
darkness	scot/o
dead body, corpse	cadaver/o
death	-mortem
death	necr/o
death	thanas/o, thanat/o
death, dead	mort/i, mort/o, mort/u
decaying, rotten	sapr/o
deep red iron-containing pigment	hem/e
deep sleep	comat/o
defecation, elimination of waste	-chezia
defective development, lack of development	aplast/o
deficiency, lack, too few	-penia
deficient, decreased	hypo-
development, formation, growth	plas/o, -plasia
development, growth, formation	plas/i, plas/o
development, nourishment	troph/o, -trophy
device that limits movement	fren/o

diaphragm, mind	phren/o
diaphragm, wall across	diaphragmat/o
digest, digestion	peps/i, -pepsia, pept/o
dilation of the pupil	mydrias/i
diluted, weakened	attenuat/o
disable	paralys/o, paralyt/o
disable	paret/o
disable	to disable
disease, sickness	morbid/o
disease, suffering, feeling, emotion	path/o, -pathy
displacement	dislocat/o
displacement	-ectopy
dissolve, separate	dilut/o
distant, far	tele/o
ditch, shallow depression	foss/o
division, split	schiz/o
double	dipl/o
down, lack of, from, not, removal	de-
down, lower, under, downward	cat-, cata-, cath-
draw back or in	retract/o
draw off, draw	spad/o
draw tightly together, bind or tie	strict/o
draw tightly together	constrict/o
dregs, sediment, waste	fec/i, fec/o
drive away	-fuge
droop, sag, prolapse, fall	-ptosis
drowsiness, oblivion	letharg/o
drug	pharmac/o, pharmaceut/o
drug, chemical	chem/i, chem/o, chemic/o
dry	kraur/o
dry	xer/o
dry, scaly	ichthy/o
drying	desic/o
dull, dim	ambly/o
duodenum	duoden/i, duoden/o
dura mater	dur/o
dusky	phe/o
dust	coni/o
dying	moribund/o

E

ear condition	-otia
ear, hearing, the sense of hearing	aud-, audi/o, audit/o
ear, hearing	aur/i, aur/o
ear, hearing	ot/o

early, premature	precoc/i
eat, swallow	phag/o
eating sore, gangrene	gangren/o
eating, swallowing	-phagia
egg	o/o, oo/o
egg	ovul/o
egg, ovum	ov/i, ov/o
elbow	cubit/o
elbow, olecranon	olecran/o
electricity, electric	electr/o
embryonic, immature, formative element	-blast
empty out	evacu/o, evacuat/o
end, limit	termin/o
enlargement	-megaly
entrance or passage	introit/o
entrance, vestibule	vestibul/o
enzyme	-ase
epididymis	epididym/o
epiglottis	epiglott/o
epithelium	epithel/i, epitheli/o
equal	iso-
esophagus	esophag/o
excessive, increased	hyper-
excessive pain, seizure, attack of severe pain	-agra
excessive, through	per-
expel from the body	eliminat/o
expose to air, fan	ventilat/o
external ear, auricle	pinn/i
extreme	pol/o
extremities (hands and feet), top, extreme point	acr/o
extremity, outermost	extrem/o, extremit/o
eye	ocul/o
eye, vision	ophthalm/o
eye, vision	opt/i, opt/o, optic/o
eyelashes, microscopic hairlike projections	cili/o
eyelid	blephar/o
eyelid	palpebr/o

F

face, form	faci/o
fall downward, slide forward	prolaps/o
falling together, symptom	symptomat/o
false	pseud/o
far	dist/o
fascia, fibrous band	fasci/o
fast, rapid	tachy-
fat	adip/o

fat, lipid	lipid/o, lip/o
fat, lipid, sebum	steat/o
feeling, nervous sensation, sense of perception	esthet/o
feeling, sensation	sens/i
female	estr/o
femur, thigh bone	femor/o
fertile, fruitful, productive	fertil/o
fertilized ovum, embryo	embry/o
fetus, unborn child	fet/i, fet/o
fever	febr/i
fever, fire	pyr/o, pyret/o, pyrex/o
fiber	fibr/o
fibrin, fibers, threads of a clot	fibrin/o
fibrous connective tissue	fibros/o
fibula	fibul/o
fibula	perone/o
field of medicine, healing	-iatrics
field of medicine	-iatry
filled in, stuffed	infarct/o
filter, to strain through	filtr/o, filtrat/o
fine tremor or shaking	tremul/o
finger or toe	digit/o
fingernail or toenail	onych/o
fingers, toes	dactyl/o
first	primi-
first	prot/o, prote/o
flame colored	flamme/o
flame within, set on fire	inflammat/o
flashing or shining forth	eclamps/o, eclampt/o
flat	plan/o
flat plate or patch	plac/o
flatus, breaking wind, rectal gas	flat/o
flesh, connective tissue	sarc/o
flood or gush back	regurgit/o
flow	flu/o
flushed, redness	erythem/o, erythemat/o
focus, point	foc/o
fold or ridge	plic/o
follicle, small sac	follicul/o
foot	pod/o
force or throw in	inject/o
forehead, brow	front/o
foreskin, prepuce	preputi/o
forking, branching	furc/o
formation, to make	-poiesis
formative material of cells	-plasm

form pus	suppur/o, suppurat/o
four	quadr/i, quadr/o
four	tetra-
free from waste, clear	defec/o, defecat/o
fringe	fimbri/o
from front to back, at the middle	midsagitt/o
from the outside, contained outside	extrins/o
full of, pertaining to, sugar	-ose
fungus	myc/e, myc/o, fung/i
funnel	infundibul/o
furnish with a mouth or outlet, new opening	-stomosis, -stomy
furrow, groove	sulc/o
furunculus, a boil, an infection	furuncul/o

G

gallbladder	cholecyst/o
ganglion	gangli/o, ganglion/o
gasping, choking	asthmat/o
gastrocnemius, calf muscle	gastrocnemi/o
gate, door	port/i
genetic change	mut/a
giant, very large	gigant/o
gingival tissue, gums	gingiv/o
give birth	-para
give up, let go, relax	remiss/o
gland	aden/o
glans penis	balan/o
glass	silic/o
glassy, made of glass	vitre/o
glomerulus	glomerul/o
glucose, sugar	gluc/o
glucose, sugar	glyc/o, glycos/o
glue	coll/a
glycogen, animal starch	glycogen/o
gnawing worm, ringworm	tine/o
go	-grade
goad, prick, incite	stimul/o
going forth	process/o
goiter, enlargement of the thyroid gland	goitr/o
gonad, sex glands	gonad/o
good, normal, well, easy	eu-
gradual impairment, breakdown, diminished function	degenerat/o
granule(s)	granul/o
gray	glauc/o
gray matter of brain and spinal cord	poli/o

great, large	magn/o
great or large toe	halluc/o
Greek letter delta, triangular shape	delt/o
green	chlor/o
grind	brux/o
groin	inguin/o
grow	-physis
grow old	senesc/o
growth, development, mold	plast/o
growth, tumor	kel/o

H

habit	-hexia
hair	pil/i, pil/o, trich/o
hair removal	depilat/o
hairy, rough	hirsut/o
half	demi-, hemi-, semi-
hallucination, to wander in the mind	hallucin/o
hand	cheir/o, chir/o, man/i, man/o
handle	manubri/o
hang	pend/o
hard	scirrh/o
hard, hardened and thickened	call/i, callos/o
hardened	indurat/o
harsh sound	strid/o
having borne one or more children	-parous
head	capit/o, cephal/o, -ceps
healthful	hygien/o
hearing, sense of hearing	acust/o, -acusia, -acusis, -cusis
hearing, sound	acous/o, acoust/o
heart	cardi/o, card/o cordi/o
heat	calor/i, therm/o
heat, burn	cauter/o, caut/o
heavy, thick	pachy-
hemoglobin	hemoglobin/o
hernia, tumor, swelling	herni/o, -cele
hidden	crypt/o
hidden, concealed	occult/o
hilum, notch or opening from a body part	hil/o
hip, hip joint	cox/o
hold back	isch/o
hold back	retent/o
holding fast, sticky	tenac/i
hollow	concav/o

hollow, cave	cav/i, cav/o
hollow, sinus	sin/o, sin/u
honey, honeyed	mellit/o
hormone	hormon/o, -one
horn, hardness	kera-
horny, hard, cornea	kerat/o
humerus (upper arm bone)	humer/o
hundred	cent-
husk, peel, bark	lemm/o
hydrochloric acid	chlorhydr/o
hymen, a membrane	hymen/o

I

ileum, small intestine	ile/o
ilium, hip bone	ili/o
immune, protection, safe	immun/o
implant, introduce	inocul/o
in	em-, ir-
in front, belly side of body	ventr/o
in, within, inside	en-, end-, endo-, in-
incomplete, imperfect	atel/o
incubation, hatching	incubat/o
infected pimple	pustul/o
infected, tainted	infect/o
infection, partition	seps/o, sept/o
infection, unclean, touching of something	contagi/o
inflammation	-itis
inherited, inheritance	hered/o, heredit/o
injury	traumat/o
innermost	intim/o
insert, send down	cathet/o
instrument for crushing	-trite
instrument for visual examination	-scope
instrument to cut	-tome
instrument used for recording	-graph
insulin	insulin/o
intense pain, agony	excruciat/o
intensive cough	pertuss/i
intestine	intestin/o
inward	eso-
iodine	iod/o
ion, to wander	ion/o
iris, choroid, ciliary body, uveal tract	uve/o
iris, colored part of eye	ir/i, ir/o, irid/o, irit/o
iron	sider/o
irregularity	anomal/o
irrigation, washing	-clysis

ischium	ischi/o
island	insul/o
itching	prurit/o

J

jaundice	icter/o
jaw	gnath/o
jejunum	jejun/o
joined together	zygot/o
joining together, linking	copulat/o
joint	arthr/o
joint	articul/o

K

ketones, acetones	ket/o, keton/o
kidney	nephr/o, ren/o
knot, swelling	nod/o
knowledge, to know	-gnosia
knuckle, knob	condyl/o

L

labor, birth	toc/o, -tocia, -tocin
lacrimal sac (tear sac)	dacryocyst/o
lamina	lamin/o
large, abnormal size or length, long	macro-
large, great	mega-
larger	major/o
largest, greatest	maxim/o
larynx, throat	laryng/o
laugh	ris/o
law, control	nom/o
layer	strat/i
lead, carry	duct/o
lead forward, yield, produce	product/o
leaven	enzym/o
left, left side	sinistr/o
lens of eye	phac/o, phak/o
less, meiosis	mei/o
lessening in density, porous condition	-porosis
life	bio-, vit/a, vit/o, viv/l
ligament	ligament/o syndesm/o
light	actin/o, lumin/o phot/o
like, resembling	-oid

limping	claudicat/o
lip	cheil/o, labi/o
listen	auscult/o
little ball	globul/o
little body	corpuscul/o
little box	capsul/o
little bundle	fascicul/o
little coil	spirill/o
little knot, swelling	tubercul/o
little knot	nodul/o
little nucleus, nucleolus	nucleol/o
little, small	-ole
liver	hepat/o
lobe, well-defined part of an organ	lob/i, lob/o
localized dilatation of the wall of a blood vessel	aneurysm/o
long-lived, long life	longev/o
look at, a kind or sort	spec/i
loosen, relax	lax/o, laxat/o
loosened, dissolved	solut/o, solv/o
louse (singular), lice (plural)	pedicul/o
lower back, loin	lumb/o
lower part of body, tail	caud/o
luminous, glowing	fluor/o
lung	pulm/o, pulmon/o
lung, air	pneum/o, pneumon/o
lying down	decubit/o
lying on the back	supin/o
lymph gland	lymphaden/o
lymph vessel	lymphangi/o
lymph, lymphatic tissue	lymph/o

M

madness, rage	man/i, rabi/o
make flow	-gog, -gogue
make soft, soften	emolli/o
make, to treat	-ize
making, producing, forming	-fic, fic/o
making, producing	-facient, -ific
malformed fetus, monster	terat/o
malleolus, little hammer	malleol/o
malleus, hammer	malle/o
mandible, lower jaw	mandibul/o
many, much	multi-, poly-
marketplace	agor/a
masculine, manly	viril/o
mastoid process	mastoid/o
maternal, or a mother	matern/o

maxilla (upper jaw)	maxill/o
maze, labyrinth, the inner ear	labyrinth/o
meal	cib/o, prandi/o, -prandial
measure	-metry
measure, instrument used to measure	-meter
mediastinum, middle	mediastin/o
medication, healing	medicat/o
medicine, physician, healing	medic/o
medulla (inner section), middle, soft, marrow	medull/o
membrane	diphther/o
membrane, thin skin	membran/o
membranes, meninges	mening/o, meningi/o
meniscus, crescent	menisc/o
menstruate, menstruation, menses	mens/o
menstruation, menses	men/o
mesentery	mesenter/o
metacarpals, bones of the hand	metacarp/o
middle	medi/o, mes-, meso-, mid-
middle, median plane	mesi/o
midwife, one who stands to receive	obstetr/i, obstetr/o
milk	galact/o, lact/i, lact/o
mimic, copy	-mimetic
mind	psych/o, -thymia
mind, chin	ment/o
mineral	mineral/o
mirror	specul/o
miter having two points on top	mitr/o
mixture of blending	-crasia
moon	lun/o, lunat/o
more, many	ple/o
motion	-kinesis
motion, movement	mot/o, motil/o
mouth	stomat/o
mouth, bone	os-
mouth, oral cavity	or/o
move, go, step, walk	grad/i
movement	kines/o, kinesi/o, -kinesia
mucuc	myx/o, myxa-
mucus	muc/o, mucos/o
muscle	muscul/o
muscle	my/o, myos/o
muscle tumor	myom/o
muscular twitching	fibrill/o
myocardium, heart muscle	myocardi/o

N

nail	ungu/o
narrow pass, throat	fauc/i
narrowing	-constriction, stric-
narrowing, contracted	sten/o
nature	physi/o, physic/o
nausea, seasickness	nause/o
navel	umbilic/o
near	proxim/o
neck	trachel-
neck, cervix (neck of uterus)	cervic/o
negative, apart, absence of	dis-
neither, neutral	neutr/o
nerve root	radicul/o
nerve, nerve tissue	nerv/o, neur/i, neur/o
nettle, rash, hives	urtic/o
network	reticul/o
neurologic tissue, supportive tissue of nervous system	gli/o
new, strange	neo-
next	nid/o
night	noct/i, nyct/o, nyctal/o
nipple	thel/o
nipple-like	papill/i, papill/o
nitrogen	niter-, nitro-
nitrogen compound	-amine
no, not without, away from, negative	a-, an-, non-
none	nulli-
normal or usual	norm/o
nose	nas/i, nas/o, rhin/o
nostril	nar/i
not	im-, un-
not continuous	intermitt/o
noun ending	-a, -y
nourishment, food, nourish, feed	nutri/o, nutrit/o
nucleus	nucle/o
nucleus, nut	kary/o
number, count	numer/o
numbness, stupor	narc/o

O

obese, extremely fat	obes/o
oblong, elongated	oblongat/o
obscure	-opaque
obsessive preoccupation	-mania
occurring in patches or circumscribed areas	areat/o

occurring monthly	menstru/o, menstruat/o
old	sen/i
old age	ger/i, ger/o, geront/o, presby/o, senil/o
omentum, fat	oment/o
on the outside, beyond, outside	extra-
one	uni-
one affected with paralysis	-plegic
one, single	mono-
one-thousandth	milli-
one who	-er, -or
one who measures	-metrist
open a wound	debrid/e
opening	-duct, hiat/o, -tresia
opening, foramen	foramin/o
opening or passageway	meat/o
orange-yellow, tawny	cirrh/o
orbit, bony cavity or socket	orbit/o
organ	organ/o
ossicle (small bone)	ossicul/o
other, different	heter/o
other, different from normal, reversal	all/o, all-
out of, outside, away from	es-, ex-, exo-
out, outside	ec-, ecto-
outside, outer	extern/o
ovary	oophor/o, ovari/o
overflowing, excessive	superflu/o
oxygen	ox/i, ox/o, ox/y
oxygen condition	-oxia

P

pain	-dynia
pain, painful condition	-algia
painful, pain sense	-algesia, -algesic
palate, roof of mouth	palat/o
pale, lacking or drained of color	pall/o, pallid/o
palm of the hand	palm/o
palm or sole	vol/o
pancreas	pancreat/o
paralysis, stroke	-plegia
parasite	parasit/o
parathyroid glands	parathyroid/o
parotid gland	parotid/o
partial dislocation	subluxat/o
partial or incomplete paralysis	-paresis
pass or go through	perme/o

patella, kneecap	patell/a, patell/o
peculiar to the individual or organ, one, distinct	idi/o
pelvic bone, pelvic cavity, hip	pelv/i, pelv/o
pen, pointed instrument	styl/o
penis	pen/i, phall/o
	priap/o
people, population	dem/o
perform, function	funct/o, function/o
perform, operate, work	oper/o, operat/o
perineum	perine/o
peritoneum	peritone/o
person who practices, specialist	-ist
perspiration	perspir/o
pertaining to	-ac, -al, -ar, -ary,
	-eal, -iac, -ial, -ic,
	-ical, -ine, -ior,
	-ory, -ous, -tic
pertaining to a cell	-cytic
pertaining to a horse	equin/o
pertaining to breathing	-pneic
pertaining to death, subject to death	mortal/i
pertaining to fate, death	fatal/o
pertaining to formation	-plastic
pertaining to killing	-cidal
pertaining to the mind	-thymic
phalanges, finger and toe	phalang/o
physician, treatment	iatr/o
pieces	segment/o
pigment, color	pigment/o
pillar	column/o
pimple	papul/o
pineal gland	pineal/o
pit	fove/o
pituitary gland	pituit/o, pituitar/o
place	loc/o, sit/u
place, position, location	top/o
placenta, round flat cake	placent/o
plant	phyt/o, -phyte
plaque, fatty substance	ather/o
plaque, plate, thin flat layer or scale	plak/o, -plakia
plentiful	copi/o
pleura, side of the body	pleur/o
plexus, network	plex/o
point of contact	synaps/o, synapt/o
point, pointed flap	cusp/i
point, spot	stigmat/o
poison, poisonous	tox/o, toxic/o
poison, virus	vir/o
polyp, small growth	polyp/o
pons (a part of the brain), bridge	pont/o

pore, small opening	por/o
potassium	kal/i
pour	-fusion
pour across, transfer	transfus/o
pour, juice	chym/o
pour out, spread apart	diffus/o
pouring out	effus/o
pouring out of juice	ecchym/o
powerful	potent/o
practice, pursue an occupation	pract/i, practic/o
pregnancy	-cyesis, gravid/o
pregnant	-gravida
pregnant, full of	pregn/o
premature expulsion of a nonviable fetus	abort/o
presence of stones	-lithiasis
press down	suppress/o
press down lower, pressed or sunk down	depress/o
press together, narrow	coarct/o, coarctat/o
pressed together, crowded together	constipat/o
pressing into	impress/o
pressure or pushing force, drive, urging on	impuls/o
pressure, weight	bar/o
prevention of conception	contracept/o
process of cutting	-tomy
process of making	-fication
process of recording	-graphy
process, state or quality of	-tion
produce, separate out	secret/o
produced by, birth, reproductive organs	genit/o
producing	-genous
producing, forming	gen-, gen/o, -gen
production, origin, formation	-gene
prostate gland	prostat/o
protection	-phylaxis
protein	globin/o, -globulin protein/o
pubis, part of hip bone	pub/o
pudendum	pudend/o
pull together	convuls/o
pulse	sphygm/o
pupil	cor/o, core/o, cor/o, pupill/o
purple	purpur/o
pus	pur/o, py/o
pus-filled	purul/o
pushed against, wedged against, packed	impact/o
put, place	the/o
put poison in	intoxic/o
pylorus, pyloric sphincter	pylor/o
pyramid shaped	pyramid/o

Q

quiet, calm, tranquil	tranquil/o

R

radiation, x-rays, radius (lateral lower arm bone)	radi/o
raise, lift up	lev/o, levat/o
rash	exanthemat/o
rays or radiant energy, giving off	radiat/o
recover, become strong	convalesc/o
recover, regain health	recuperat/o
rectum, straight	rect/o
red	erythr/o, rube-
red, rosy	eosin/o
reduce, destroy	-lytic
related to the male	andr/o
relating to water	hydr/o, hydra-
relationship to movement	cine-
relationship to pain	alg/e, algi/o, alg/o, algesi/o
relaxation	-chalasis, -chalasia
removal	-apheresis -pheresis
renal pelvis, bowl of kidney	pyel/o
render unclean by contact, pollute	contaminat/o
reproduce	procreat/o
reproduce, bear offspring	prolifer/o
resembling, in the shape of	-form, form/o
resulting record	-gram
retina, net	retin/o
revive	resuscit/o
rhythm	rhythm/o
rib	cost/o
right side	dextr/o
rigid, tense	tetan/o
ring or circle	circ/i
ringing, buzzing, tinkling	tinnit/o
ripe	matur/o
ripe age, adult	pubert/o
rod-shaped bacterium (plural, bacteria)	bacill/o
roll, turn	volv/o
rolled up, curled inward	involut/o
root	rhiz/o
rotate, revolve	rotat/o
rottenness, decay	cari/o
round, sphere, ball	spher/o
run, running	-drome
running ahead, precursor	prodrom/o
running together	syndrom/o
rupture	-rrhexis

S

sacx	sacc/i, sacc/o
sacrum	sacr/o
saddle	sell/o
saliva	-ptyal/o, saliv/o
	sial/o
salivary gland	sialaden/o
same	ipsi-
same, equal	is/o
same, like, alike	hom/o
sameness, unchanging, constant	home/o
scale	squam/o
scanty, few	olig/o
scapula, shoulder blade	scapul/o
scar	cicatric/o
sclera, white of eye, hard	scler/o
sea	thalass/o
seam, suture	raph/o
sebum	seb/o
secrete	crin/o, -crine
secrete milk	lactat/o
secrete out of	exocrin/o
secrete within	endocrin/o
seed	gon/e, gon/o
seed, spore	spor/o
seeing, sight	vis/o
seize, take hold of	-leptic
seizure	-lepsy
self	aut/o
semen, seed, sperm	semin/i
seminal vesicle, blister, little bladder	vesicul/o
send	-mission
sensation, feeling	-esthesia, esthesi/o
sensation, sense of perception	aesthet/o
sensitive to, affected by	sensitiv/o
separate	-crit
separate, discharge	excret/o
separation, away from, opposed, detached	ap-, apo-
serous	seros/o
serum	ser/o
sexual drive, desire, passion	libid/o, libidin/o
sexual intercourse	vener/o, -pareunia
sexual love	erot/o
shaded, dark, impenetrable to light	opac/o, opacit/o
shaken together, violently agitated	concuss/o
shaking, trembling	trem/o
shape, form	morph/o
shaped like a lens, pertaining to a lens	lenticul/o
shaped or formed like, resembling	-iform
share, to make common	communic/o

sharp, severe, sudden	acu/o
sharp, sharpness	acuit/o, acut/o
sheath	thec/o
sheath, covering	-lemma
shedding, falling off	decidu/o
shell	conch/o
short	brachy-, brev/i, brev/o
shoulder	om/o
shut, close up	occlud/o, occlus/o
shut or close	clus/o
side	later/o
sieve	ethm/o
sigmoid colon	sigmoid/o
singular noun ending	-um
sinus	sinus/o
skeleton	skelet/o
skill	techn/o, techni/o
skin	cutane/o, derma-, dermat/o, derm/o
skin spot	petechi/o
skin, leather	cori/o
skull	crani/o
slanted, sideways	obliqu/o
sleep	hypn/o, somn/i, somn/o, sopor/o
slender; thin	lept/o
slender	gracil/o
slide	lux/o
slide, fall, sag	-lapse
slip, fall, slide	laps/o
slipping	-listhesis
slow	brady-
small	micr/o, micro-
small intestine	enter/o
small, little	-ula
small one	-ule
smaller	minor/o
smaller, less	mio-
smallest, least	minim/o
smell, odor	-osmia
smell, sense of smell	olfact/o
smooth (visceral) muscle	leiomy/o
snore, snoring	rhonc/o, stert/o
socket or pit	glen/o
sodium	natr/o
sole of foot	plant/i, plant/o
solid structure	ster/o
solid, three-dimensional	stere/o

solution	-sol
something inserted or thrown in	embol/o
something molded or formed	plasm/o
sore, ulcer	ulcer/o
sound	ech/o, son/o
sound, healthy, sane	san/o
sound, voice	phon/o, -phonia
soundness, health	sanit/o
spark	scintill/o
speak or speech	-phasia, -ian,
specialist	-iatrist, -ician,
	-ologist
speech	phas/o
sperm, spermatozoa, seed	sperm/o, spermat/
sphenoid bone, wedge	sphen/o
spherical bacteria	cocc/i, cocc/o,
	-coccus
spider web, spider	arachn/o
spinal column, vertebrae	rachi/o
spinal cord, bone marrow	myel/o
spinal cord, cord	chord/o
spine, backbone	spin/o
spiny, thorny	acanth/o
spiral, snail, snail shell	cochle/o
spitting	-ptysis
spleen	splen/o
split, divided into two parts	bifid/o
split	-fida
spot	macul/o
spread out, expand	dilat/o, dilatat/o
sputum, spit	sput/o
squint, squint-eyed	strab/i
standing apart, expansion	diastol/o
stapes (middle ear bone)	staped/o, stapedi/o
star, star-shaped	astr/o
starch	amyl/o
state of	-ancy
steal	klept/o
sterile	steril/i
sternum, the breastbone	stern/o
stick to, cling to	adhes/o
sticky	visc/o, viscos/o
stiff	rigid/o
stimulate, act on	-tropin
sting, prick, puncture	punct/o
stitch, seam	sutur/o
stomach, belly	gastr/o
stone, calculus	lith/o, -lith
stone, little stone	calcul/o
stopping	-pause

straight, normal, correct	orth/o
strange, foreign	xen/o
strange, out of place	atop/o
strength	-sthenia
stretch	tone/o
stretch apart, expand	distend/o, distent/o
stretch out, extend, strain	tens/o
stretching, dilation, enlargement	ectasia, -ectasis
striated muscle	rhabdomy/o
strike, tap, beat	percuss/o
string of beads, genus of parasitic mold or fungi	monil/i
stripe, furrow, groove	striat/o
structure, tissue	-ium
study of	-logy
stupor, sleep	carot/o
substance	-in, -ine
substance that forms	-poietin
sudden attack	paroxysm/o
sudden involuntary contraction, tightening or cramping	-spasm, spasmod/o
sudden	-oxysm/o
sugar	sacchar/o, sucr/o
sulfur	thio-
surgical fixation of bone or joint, to bind, tie together	-desis
surgical fixation of vertebrae	-syndesis
surgical fixation	-pexy
surgical puncture to remove fluid	-centesis
surgical removal, cutting out, excision	-ectomy
surgical repair	-plasty
surgically creating an opening	-ostomy
surrounding, around	peri-
suture	-rrhaphy
swallow	deglutit/o
sweat	diaphor/o, hidr/o sudor/i
sweat out	exud/o, exudat/o
sweet	glycer/o
swell, be excited	orgasm/o
swelling, fluid, tumor	-dema, edem-, edemat/o
swelling	-edema
swift, sharp, acid	oxy-
sword	xiph/i, xiph/o
sympathize with	compatibil/o
synovial membrane, synovial fluid	synovi/o, synov/o
syphilis	syphil/i, syphil/o

T

take up or receive within	intussuscept/o

tarsus (ankle bone), instep, edge of the eyelid	tars/o
tasteless	insipid/o
tear, tear duct, lacrimal duct	dacry/o, lacrim/o
temporal bone, temple	tempor/o
ten, tenth	deca-, deci-
tending to increase urine output	diur/o, diuret/o
tendon	tendin/o
tendon, stretch out, extend, strain	ten/o, tend/o
tension, tone, stretching	ton/o
testicles, testis, testes	orch/o, orchid/o, orchi/o
testis, testicle	test/i, test/o, testicul/o
thalamus, inner room	thalam/o
the lens of the eye	lent/i
the nape	nuch/o
the science or study of	-ology
the space between things	interstiti/o
thick mucus	phlegm/o
thing, singular noun ending	-us
thirst	dips/o, -dipsia
three	tri-
throat	jugul/o
throat, pharynx	pharyng/o
throbbing, quivering	palpit/o
through, between, apart, complete	dia-
throw or hurl out	ejaculat/o
thumb	pollic/o
thymus gland, soul	thym/o
thyroid gland	thyr/o, thyroid/o
tibia (shin bone)	tibi/o
tight band	sphincter/o
time	chron/o
tissue	hist/o, histi/o
tissue death	-necrosis
together, with	co-, com-, con-
together, with, union, association	syn-
tongue	gloss/o, lingu/o
tonsil, throat	tonsill/o
too early, untimely	prematur/o
tooth, teeth	dent/i, dent/o, odont/o
torn, mangled	lacer/o, lacerat/o
touch	tact/i
touch, feel, stroke	palpat/o
touched, infected	contact/o
toward, to	af-, ap-, as-, at-
toward, to, in direction of	ad-
trachea, windpipe	trache/i, trache/o

treatment	therap/o, therapeut/o
trigone	trigon/o
tube	syring/o
tube, pipe	tub/i, tub/o
tube or pipe	fistul/o
tumor	onc/o
tumor, neoplasm	-oma
turn	vers/o, vert/o
turn	-verse, -version
turn, change	trop/o, -tropia
turned or twisted out	exstroph/o
turning	-tropic
turning aside	divert/i
turning point	cris/o, critic/o
turning, folding	gyr/o
twice, double, two	bi-, bis-
twice, twofold, double	di-
twin, double	gemin/o
twist, rotate	tors/o
twisted chain	strept/o
twisted	tort/i
two by two	bin-
tympanic membrane, eardrum	myring/o, tympan/o

U

ulcer	aphth/o
ulna (medial lower arm bone)	uln/o
umbilical cord, the navel	omphal/o
unable to speak, inarticulate	mut/o
under, less, below	sub-
uneasy, anxious, fearful	anxi/o, anxiet/o
unequal	anis/o
unexplained, of one's own accord	spontane/o
unnamed, nameless	innominat/o
untouched, whole	intact/o
up, apart, backward, excessive	an-, ana-
upright	erect/o
urea, nitrogen	azot/o
ureter	ureter/o
urethra	urethr/o
urinary bladder	vesic/o
urinary bladder, cyst, sac of fluid	cyst/o
urinate	mictur/o, micturit/o
urination, urine	-uria
urination	-uresis

urine or urinary organs	urin/o
urine, urinary tract	ur/o
use of hands	manipul/o
uterine (fallopian) tube, auditory (eustachian) tube	salping/o, -salpinx
uterus	hyster/o, metr/i, metr/o, metri/o
uterus	uter/i, uter/o
uvula, little grape	uvul/o

V

vaccine	vaccin/i, vaccin/o
vagina	colp/o, vagin/o
vagus nerve, wandering	vag/o
valve	valv/o, valvul/o
varicose veins, swollen or dilated vein	varic/o
varied, irregular	poikil/o
vas deferens, vessel	vas/o
vast, great, extensive	vast/o
vein	phleb/o, ven/o
ventricle of brain or heart, small chamber	ventricul/o
venule, small vein	venul/o
vertebra, backbone	vertebr/o
vertebrae, vertebral column, back bone	spondyl/o
viscera, internal organ	viscer/o
vision condition	-opia
vision, view of	-opsia, -opsis, -opsy
visual examination	-scopy
voice	voc/i
vomit	emet/o
vomiting	-emesis
vulva	episi/o
vulva, covering	vulv/o

W

walk	ambul/o, ambulat/o
wall	pariet/o
wandering in the mind	deliri/o
wart	verruc/o
wash, bathe	lav/o, lavat/o
wasted by disease	emaciat/o
wasting away	-phthisis
water	aqu/i, aqu/o, aque/o
watery flow, subject to flow	rheum/o, rheumat/o
wax	cera-
weakness, lack of strength	asthen-, asthenia

what is given	-dote
whirling round	vertig/o, vertigin/o
white	alb/i, alb/o, albin/o
	leuk/o
wide	mydri/o
widely scattered	disseminat/o
widening, stretching, expanding	-dilation
widening	-eurysm
wife or husband, sperm or egg	gamet/o
window	fenestr/o
with, together, joined together	sym-
within	ento-
within, inner	intern/o
within, inside	intra-
within, into, inside	intro-
without an opening	atres/i
without teeth	edentul/o
wolf	lup/i, lup/o
woman, female	gynce/o
work	erg/o, -ergy
worm	verm/i
worsening or gradual impairment	deteriorat/o
wrinkle	rhytid/o
wrinkle, fold	rug/o
wrist bones	carp/o
write	scrib/o, script/o

X

x-ray	roentgen/o

Y

yellow	lute/o, xanth/o
yellow; jaundice	jaund/o

SECTION 3

Common Abbreviations and Meanings

■ ■ ■

A

a	before
A2 or A_2	aortic valve closure
A	accommodation; age; anterior
AAA	abdominal aortic aneurysm
AAL	anterior axillary line
Ab	antibody
AB, ab	abortion
AB	abnormal
A/B	acid–base ratio
ABC	aspiration; biopsy; cytology
abd	abdomen
ABE	acute bacterial endocarditis
ABG	arterial blood gases
ABP	arterial blood pressure
AC	acromioclavicular; air conduction
ac	acute
AC, ac	before meals
Acc	accommodation
ACD	acid-citrate-dextrose; anterior chest diameter
ACE	angiotensin-converting enzyme
ACG	angiocardiography; apex cardiogram
ACH	adrenocortical hormone
ACL	anterior cruciate ligament
ACLS	advanced cardiac life support
ACP	acid phosphatase
ACTH	adrenocorticotropic hormone
ACVD	acute cardiovascular disease
AD	abdominal diaphragmatic breathing; adenovirus; Alzheimer's disease; right ear
ADD	attention deficit disorder
ADE	adverse drug event

ADH	antidiuretic hormone
ADHD	attention deficit hyperactivity disorder
ADL	activities of daily living
ad lib	as desired
adm	admission
ADS	antibody deficiency syndrome
ADR	adverse drug reaction
ADT	admission; discharge; transfer
AE	above elbow
AED	automated external defibrillation
AF	acid-fast; atrial fibrillation
AFB	acid-fast bacilli
A fib	atrial fibrillation
AFP	alpha-fetoprotein
Ag	antigen
AG, A/G	albumin/globulin ratio
AH	abdominal hysterectomy
AHD	arteriosclerotic heart disease; autoimmune hemolytic disease
AHF	antihemophilic factor VIII
AHG	antihemophilic globulin factor VIII
AI	aortic insufficiency; atherogenic index
AID	acute infectious disease; artificial insemination donor
AIDS	acquired immune deficiency syndrome
AIH	artificial insemination homologous
AIHA	autoimmune hemolytic anemia
aj	ankle jerk
AK	above knee
AKA	above-knee amputation; also known as
alb	albumin
ALG	antilymphocytic globulin
alk	alkaline
alk phos	alkaline phosphatase
ALL	acute lymphoblastic leukemia; acute lymphocytic leukemia
ALP	alkaline phosphatase
ALS	aldolase; amyotrophic lateral sclerosis; antilymphocytic serum
ALT	alanine transaminase (liver and heart enzyme)
alt dieb	alternate days; every other day
alt hor	alternate hours
alt noct	alternate nights
AMA	advanced maternal age; against medical advice; American Medical Association
amb	ambulate; ambulatory
AMD	age-related macular degeneration
AMI	acute myocardial infarction
AML	acute myeloblastic leukemia; acute myelocytic leukemia
amp	ampule
AMS	amylase

amt	amount
AN	anesthesiology
ANA	antinuclear antibodies
ANF	antinuclear factor
ANLL	acute nonlymphocytic leukemia
ANS	autonomic nervous system
ant	anterior
AOD	adult-onset diabetes; arterial occlusive disease
AOM	acute otitis media
A & P	anterior and posterior; auscultation and percussion
AP	angina pectoris; anteroposterior; anterior-posterior
APLD	aspiration percutaneous lumbar diskectomy
aq	aqueous; water
ARD	acute respiratory disease
ARDS	adult respiratory distress syndrome
ARF	acute renal failure; acute respiratory failure
ARM	artificial rupture of membranes
ART	assisted reproductive technology
AS	ankylosing spondylitis; aortic stenosis; left ear
ASA	aspirin
ASAP	as soon as possible
ASCVD	arteriosclerotic cardiovascular disease
ASD	atrial septal defect
ASH	asymmetrical septal hypertrophy
ASHD	arteriosclerotic heart disease
ASIS	anterior superior iliac spine
ASO	arteriosclerosis obliterans
ASS	anterior superior spine
AST	aspartate aminotransferase
as tol	as tolerated
ATP	adenosine triphosphate
Au	gold
AU	aures unitas (both ears)
AUL	acute undifferentiated leukemia
ausc	auscultation
A-V	aortic valve; artificial ventilation; atrioventricular; arteriovenous
AVM	arteriovenous malfunction
AVN	atrioventricular node
AVR	aortic valve replacement
Ax	axillary
AZT	Aschheim-Zondek test

B

B/A	backache
BA	bronchial asthma
Ba	barium
BAC	blood alcohol concentration
BaE	barium enema
BAO	basal acid output

bas	basophils
BBB	blood–brain barrier; bundle branch block
BBT	basal body temperature
BC	bone conduction
BCC	basal cell carcinoma
BE	barium enema; below elbow
BEAM	brain electrical activity map
BED	binge eating disorder
BFP	biologic false positive
BID, bid, b.i.d.	bis in die; twice a day
bil	bilateral
BIN, bin	twice a night
BK	below knee
BKA	below-knee amputation
Bld	blood
BJ	Bence Jones
BM	bone marrow; bowel movement
BMD	Becker's muscular dystrophy; bone mineral density
BMI	body mass index
BMR	basal metabolic rate
BMT	barium meal test; bone marrow transplant
BNO	bladder neck obstruction
BNR	bladder neck resection
BOM	bilateral otitis media
B/P, BP	blood pressure
BP&P	blood pressure and pulse
BPH	benign prostatic hyperplasia; benign prostatic hypertrophy
BPM, bpm	beats per minute; breaths per minute
BPPV	benign paroxysmal positional vertigo
BR	bedrest
BRBPR	bright red blood per rectum (hematochochezia)
Bronch	bronchoscopy
BRP	bathroom privileges
BS	blood sugar; bowel sounds; breath sounds
BSE	breast self-examination
BSO	bilateral salpingo-oophorectomy
BT	bleeding time
BUN	blood urea nitrogen
BV	bacterial vaginosis; blood volume
Bx, bx	biopsy

C

C_1 through C_7	cervical vertebrae
C	centigrade; Celsius
c	centimeter
$\bar{c}$	with
$\underline{c}$	without
Ca	calcium
CA, Ca	cancer; cardiac arrest; carcinoma; chronological age

CAB	coronary artery bypass
CABG	coronary artery bypass grafting
CAD	computer-assisted diagnosis; coronary artery disease
cal	calorie
cap, caps	capsule
CAPD	continuous ambulatory peritoneal dialysis
CAT	computerized axial tomography
cath	catheter; catheterize
CAVH	continuous arteriovenous hemofiltration
CBC, cbc	complete blood count
CBF	capillary blood flow; coronary blood flow
CBI	continuous bladder irrigation
CBR	complete bedrest
CBS	chronic brain syndrome
CC	chief complaint; colony count; cardiac cycle; creatinine clearance; cardiac catheterization
cc	cubic centimeter (1/1000 liter)
CCA	circumflex coronary artery
CCCR	closed chest cardiopulmonary resuscitation
CCPD	continuous cycle peritoneal dialysis
CCr	creatinine clearance
CCT	cranial computed tomography
CCU	coronary care unit
CDC	calculated date (day) of confinement; Centers for Disease Control and Prevention
CDE	common duct exploration
CDH	congenital dislocation of the hip
CDT	cumulative trauma disorders
CEA	carcinoembryonic antigen
CF	complete fixation; counting fingers; cystic fibrosis
CFS	chronic fatigue syndrome
C gl	with correction; with glasses
CGL	chronic granulomatous leukemia
CHB	complete heart block
CHD	congenital heart defects; coronary heart disease
CHF	congestive heart failure
CHO	carbohydrate
chol	cholesterol
chr	chronic
CI	coronary insufficiency
cib	food
CID	cytomegalic inclusion disease
CIE	counter-immunoelectrophoresis
CIN	cervical intraepithelial neoplasia
circ	circumcision
CIS	carcinoma in situ
CIT	conventional insulin treatment
CK	creatine kinase
ck	check
Cl, cl	clinic; chloride

CL	cholelithiasis; chronic leukemia; cirrhosis of the liver; cleft lip; corpus luteum
CLD	chronic liver disease
CLL	chronic lymphocytic leukemia
cl liq	clear liquid
cm	centimeter (1/100 meter)
cm^3	cubic centimeter
CME	cystoid macular edema
CMG	cystometrogram
CML	chronic myelocytic leukemia
CMM	cutaneous malignant melanoma
CMV	controlled mechanical ventilation; cystometrogram; cytomegalovirus
CNS	central nervous system; cutaneous nerve stimulation
c/o	complains of
Co	cobalt
CO	carbon monoxide; coronary occlusion; coronary output
CO$_2$	carbon dioxide
COLD	chronic obstructive lung disease
comp	compound
cond	condition
contra	against
COPD	chronic obstructive pulmonary disease
CP	cardiopulmonary; cerebral palsy
CPA	carotid phonoangiograph
CPAP	continuous positive airway pressure
CPC	clinicopathologic conference
CPD	cephalopelvic disproportion
CPE	cytopathic effect
CPK	creatine phosphokinase
CPN	chronic pyelonephritis
CPPB	continuous positive-pressure breathing
CPR	cardiopulmonary resuscitation
CPS	cycles per second
CRD	chronic respiratory disease
CRF	chronic renal failure
creat	creatinine
CR	conditioned reflex; complete response
CRF	chronic renal failure
CS	central supply; cesarean section; complete stroke; conditioned stimulus; Cushing's syndrome
C & S	culture and sensitivity
C-section	cesarean section
CSAP	cryosurgical ablation of the prostate
CSF	cerebrospinal fluid
C-spine	cervical spine (films)
CSR	central supply room; Cheyne-Stokes respiration
CT	computed tomography
CTCL	cutaneous T-cell lymphoma
CTS	carpal tunnel syndrome

CTT	computed transaxial tomography
CTZ	chemoreceptor trigger zone
cu	cubic
CUC	chronic ulcerative colitis
CUG	cystourethrogram
CV	cardiovascular
CVA	cardiovascular accident; cerebrovascular accident; costovertebral angle
CVD	cardiovascuascular disease
CVL	central venous line
CVP	central venous pressure; Cytoxan, vincristine, prednisone
CVS	chorionic villus sampling
CWP	childbirth without pain; coal workers' pneumoconiosis
Cx	cervix
CX, CXR	chest x-ray film
cysto	cystoscopic examination; cystoscopy

D

D	diopter (lens strength)
d	day
DAT	diet as tolerated
db	decibel
D & C	dilation and curettage
D/C, DC	discontinue
DCC	direct-current cardioversion
DCIS	ductal carcinoma in situ
DCR	direct cortical response
D & E	dilation and evacuation
del	delivery
DES	diethylstilbestrol
DGE	delayed gastric emptying
DEXA	dual energy x-ray absorptiometry
DHEA	dehydroepiandrosterone
DHFS	dengue hemorrhagic fever shock syndrome
DI	diabetes insipidus
diag	diagnosis
DIC	diffuse intravascular coagulation
diff	differential
DIP	distal interphalangeal
disch	discharge
DJD	degenerative joint disease
DKA	diabetic ketoacidosis
DLE	discoid lupus erythematosus
DM	dermatomyositis; diabetes mellitus; diastolic murmur
DMD	Duchenne's muscular dystrophy
DNA	deoxyribonucleic acid
DNR	do not resuscitate
DNS	deviated nasal septum
D.O.	Doctor of Osteopathy
DOA	dead on arrival

DOB	date of birth
DOE	dyspnea on exertion
DOMS	delayed-onset muscle soreness
DOT	directly observed therapy
DQ	developmental quotient
DPT	diphtheria-pertussis-tetanus
dr	dram; dressing
DR	diabetic retinopathy
DR	digital radiography; doctor
DRG	diagnosis-related group
D/S	dextrose in saline
DSA	digital subtraction angiography
DSD	dry sterile dressing
dsg	dressing
DT	diphtheria and tetanus toxoids
DTP	diphtheria, tetanus toxoids, and pertussis vaccine
DTs	delirium tremens
DTR	deep tendon reflex
DUB	dysfunctional uterine bleeding
DVA	distance visual acuity
DVI	digital vascular imaging
DVT	deep vein thrombosis
DW	distilled water
D/W	dextrose in water
Dx	diagnosis

E

E	enema
EBL	estimated blood loss
EBP	epidural blood patch
EBV	Epstein-Barr virus
ECC	endocervical curettage; extracorporeal circulation
ECCE	extracapsular lens extraction
ECG	electrocardiogram; electrocardiography
ECHO	echocardiogram; eccardiography
ECMO	extracorporeal membrane oxygenation
ECT	electroconvulsive therapy
ED	effective dose; emergency department
EDC	estimated date (day) of confinement
EDD	end-diastolic dimension
EDG	electrodynogram
EDV	end-diastolic volume
EEG	electroencephalogram; electroencephalography
EENT	eye, ear, nose, and throat
EFM	electronic fetal monitor
EIA	enzyme immunoassay
EIB	exercise-induced bronchospasm
Ej	elbow jerk
EKG	electrocardiogram; electrocardiography

ELISA	enzyme-linked immunoassay; enzyme-linked immunosorbent assay
elix	elixir
EM	electron microscope; emmetropia
EMG	electromyogram; electromyography
EMR	educable mentally retarded; electronic medical record; eye movement record
EMS	early morning specimen; electromagnetic spectrum
ENG	electronystagmography
ENT	ear, nose, and throat
EOG	electro-oculogram
EOM	extraocular muscles; extraocular movement
Eos, eosins	eosinophils
EP	ectopic pregnancy; evoked potential
EPF	early pregnancy factor; exophthalmos-producing factor
EPO	erythropoietin
EPR	electron paramagnetic resonance; emergency physical restraint
EPS	extrapyramidal symptoms; exophthalmos-producing substance
ER	emergency room; epigastric region
ERCP	endoscopic retrograde cholangiopancreatography
ERG	electroretinogram
ERPF	effective renal plasma flow
ERT	estrogen replacement therapy; external radiation therapy
ERV	expiratory reserve volume
ESD	end-systolic dimension
ESPF	end-stage pulmonary fibrosis
ESR	erythrocyte sedimentation rate
ESRD	end-stage renal disease
ESWL	extracorporeal shock-wave lithotripsy
EST	electric shock therapy
ESV	end-systolic volume
ET	embryo transfer; enterically transmitted; esotropia
et	and
ETF	eustachian tube function
etiol	etiology
ETT	endotracheal tube; exercise tolerance test
EU	Ehrlich units; emergency unit; etiology unknown
EWB	estrogen withdrawal bleeding
ex	excision; exercise
exam	examination
exp	expiration
ext	extraction; external

F

F	Fahrenheit
FA	fluorescent antibody
FAS	fetal alcohol syndrome

FB	foreign body
FBS	fasting blood sugar
FCD	fibrocystic disease
FDA	Food and Drug Administration
FDP	fibrin-fibrinogen degradation products
Fe	iron
FECG	fetal electrocardiogram
FEF	forced expiratory flow
FEV	forced expiratory volume
FFA	free fatty acids
FH	family history
FHR	fetal heart rate
FHS	fetal heart sounds
FHT	fetal heart tones
FIA	fluorescent immunoassay; fluoroimmunoassay
FME	full mouth extractions
FMS	fibromyalgia syndrome
FOBT	fecal occult blood test
FPG	fasting plasma glucose
FR	fibrin-fibrinogen related
fr	French (catheter size)
FRC	functional residual capacity
FROM	full range of motion
FS	frozen section
FSH	follicle-stimulating hormone
FSP	fibrin-fibrinogen split products
FSS	funnctional endoscopic sinus surgery
FT	family therapy
FTA	fluorescent treponemal antibody
FTI	free thyroxine index
FTND	full-term normal delivery
FTT	failure to thrive
FU	follow-up; follow up
FUO	fever of unknown origin
FX, Fx	fracture

G

g	gram
g_1	gravida (pregnancy)
Ga	gallium
GA	gastric analysis; general anesthesia
GB	gallbladder
GBM	glomerular basement membrane
GBS	gallbladder series; Guillain-Barré syndrome
G-Cs	glucocorticoids
GC	gonorrhea
GDM	gestational diabetes mellitus
GER	gastroesophageal reflux
GERD	gastroesophageal reflux disease

GFR	glomerular filtration rate
GG	gamma globulin
GGT	gamma-glutamyl transferase
GH	growth hormone
GHb	glycohemoglobin
GIFT	gamete intrafallopian transfer
GIT	gastrointestinal tract
GLTT	glucose tolerance test
gm	gram
GMP	guanosine monophosphate
GOT	glutamic oxaloacetic transaminase
GP	general practice
gr	grain
grav I	pregnancy one; primigravida
GS	general surgery
GSW	gunshot wound
gt	drop
GTP	guanosine triphosphate
GTT	glucose tolerance test
gtt	drops
GU	genitourinary
GVHD	graft-versus-host disease
GxT	graded exercise test
GYN, Gyn	gynecology

H

h	hour
H	hydrogen; hypodermic
H_2 blocker	H_2 receptor antagonist
H & H	hemoglobin and hematocrit
HAA	hepatitis associated antigen; hepatitis Australia antigen
HAI	hemagglutination-inhibition immunoassay
HASHD	hypertensive arteriosclerotic heart disease
HAV	hepatitis A virus
HB	heart block; hemoglobin
HBE	His bundle electrocardiogram
HbF	fetal hemoglobin
HBP	high blood pressure
HbS	sickle cell hemoglobin
HBV	hepatitis B virus
HC	Huntington's chorea
HCFA	Health Care Financing Administration
HCG, hCG	human chorionic gonadotropin
HCl	hydrochloric acid
HCL	hairy cell leukemia
HCPCS	Health Care Financing Administration Common Procedure Coding System
HCT, hct	hematocrit
HCV	hepatitis C virus

HCVD	hypertensive cardiovascular disease
HD	hearing distance; heart disease; hemodialysis; hip disarticulation; Hodgkin's disease; Huntington's disease
HDL	high-density lipoprotein
He	helium
H & E	hematoxylin and eosin stain
HDN	hemolytic disease of the newborn
HDS	herniated disk syndrome
HE	hereditary elliptocytosis
HEENT	head, eyes, ears, nose, throat
HF	heart failure
Hg	mercury
HgA$_{1c}$	glycohemoglobin test
Hgb	hemoglobin
HGE	human granulocytic Ehrlichiosis
HI	hemagglutination-inhibition
HIE	hypoxic ischemic encephalopathy
HIV	human immunodeficiency virus
H & L	heart and lungs
HL	Hodgkin's lymphoma
HLA	human leukocyte antigen
HLR	heart-lung resuscitation
HM	hand motion
HMD	hyaline membrane disease
HMO	health maintenance organization
HNP	herniated nucleus pulposus
HO	hyperbaric oxygen
h/o	history of
HOB	head of bed
H$_2$O	water
H & P	history and physical
HP	hemipelvectomy; hyperparathyroidism
HPF	high-power field
HPL	human placental lactogen
HPO	hypothalamic-pituitary-ovarian
HPS	hantavirus pulmonary syndrome
HPV	human papilloma virus
HR	heart rate
hr	hour
HRT	hormone replacement therapy
hs, h.s.	at bedtime; hour of sleep
HS	hereditary spherocytosis; herpes simplex
HSG	hysterosalpingogram
HSV	herpes simplex virus
ht	height; hematocrit; hormone therapy
HTO	high tibial osteotomy
HTN	hypertension
HV	hospital visit
HVD	hypertensive vascular disease
Hx	history

hypo	hypodermic
HZ	herpes zoster
I	
I	intensity of magnetism; iodine
IABP	intra-aortic balloon pump
IACP	intra-aortic counterpulsation
IADH	inappropriate antidiuretic hormone
IASD	interatrial septal defect
IBC	iron-binding capacity
IBD	inflammatory bowel disease
IBS	irritable bowel syndrome
IC	inspiratory capacity
ICCE	intracapsular lens extraction
ICCU	intensive coronary care unit
ICF	intracellular fluid
ICP	intracranial pressure
ICS	intercostal space
ICSI	intracytoplasmic sperm injection
ICT	indirect Coombs' test; insulin coma therapy
ict ind	icterus index
ICU	intensive care unit
I & D	incision and drainage
ID	infectious disease; intradermal
IDC	infiltrating ductal carcinoma; invasive ductal carcinoma
IDD	insulin-dependent diabetes
IDDM	insulin-dependent diabetes mellitus
IDK	internal derangement of the knee
IDS	immunity deficiency state
I/E	inspiratory-expiratory ratio
IEMG	integrated electromyogram
IFG	impaired fasting glucose
Ig	immunoglobulin
IgA	immunoglobulin A
IgD	immunoglobulin D
IgE	immunoglobulin E
IgG	immunoglobulin G
IgM	immunoglobulin M
IGT	impaired glucose tolerance
IH	infectious hepatitis
IHD	ischemic heart disease
IHSS	idiopathic hypertrophic subaortic stenosis
IL	interleukin
ILC	infiltrating lobar carcinoma; invasive lobular carcinoma
IM	infectious mononucleosis; intramuscular
IMAG	internal mammary artery graft
IMF	idiopathic myelofibrosis
IMV	intermittent mandatory ventilation
inf	inferior; infusion
INH	isoniazid

I & O	intake and output
IO	intraocular
IOD	iron-overload disease (hemochromatosis)
IOL	intraocular lens
IOP	intraocular pressure
IPF	idiopathic pulmonary fibrosis
IPG	impedance plethysmography
IPPB	intermittent positive-pressure breathing
IQ	intelligence quotient
irrig	irrigation
IS	intercostal space
ISG	immune serum globulin
isol	isolation
ITP	idiopathic thrombocytopenic purpura
IU	international unit
IUD	intrauterine device
IUP	intrauterine pressure
IV	intravenous; intravenously
IVC	inferior vena cava
IVCP	inferior vena cava pressure
IVD	intervertebral disk
IVDA	intravenous drug abuse
IVF	in vitro fertilization
IVFA	intravenous fluorescein angiography
IVP	intravenous pyelogram
IVSD	interventricular septal defect
IVU	intravenous urogram

J

jct	junctions
JOD	juvenile-onset diabetes
JRA	juvenile rheumatoid arthritis
Jt	joint
JVP	jugular venous pressure; jugular venous pulse

K

K	potassium
KB	ketone bodies
KCF	key clinical findings
KCl	potassium chloride
KD	knee disarticulation
KE	kinetic energy
kg	kilogram
kj	knee jerk
KO	keep open
KOH	potassium hydrochloride
KS	Kaposi's sarcoma
KUB	kidney, ureter, bladder
KVO	keep vein open

L

l, L	liter
L_1–L_5	lumbar vertebrae
L & A	light and accommodation
LA	left atrium
lab	laboratory
lac	laceration
LAD	left anterior descending
LAP	leucine aminopeptidase
lap	laparotomy
laser	light amplification by stimulated emission of radiation
LASIK	laser in situ keratomileusis
lat	lateral
LAVH	laparoscopically assisted vaginal hysterectomy
lb	pound
LB	large bowel; low back
LBBB	left bundle branch block
LBW	low birth weight
LBBX	left breast biopsy and examination
LBP	low back pain
LCIS	lobular carcinoma in situ
L & D	labor and delivery
LD	lactic dehydrogenase
LDD	light-dark discrimination
LDH	lactic dehydrogenase
LDL	low-density lipoprotein
LE	life expectancy; lower extremity; lupus erythematosus
LEEP	loop electrocautery excision procedure
LES	lower esophageal sphincter
lg	large
LH	luteinizing hormone
LHBD	left heart bypass device
LHF	left-sided heart failure
LHR	leukocyte histamine release test
lig	ligament
liq	liquid
L K & S	liver, kidney, and spleen
LLE	lower left extremity
LLL	left lower lobe
LLSB	left lower sternal border
LLQ	left lower quadrant
L/min	liters per minute
LMP	last menstrual period
LNMP	last normal menstrual period
LOC	level of consciousness; loss of consciousness
LOM	limitation of motion; loss of motion
LOS	length of stay
LP	light perception; lumbar puncture; lumboperitoneal
LPF	low-power field

LPS	lipase
LR	light reaction
LRDKT	living related donor kidney transplant
LSB	left sternal border
LSD	lysergic acid diethylamide
lt	left
LTB	laryngotracheobronchitis
LTC	long-term care
LTH	luteotropic hormone
LUE	left upper extremity
LUL	left upper lobe
LUQ	left upper quadrant
LV	left ventricle
LVH	left ventricle hypertrophy
lymphs	lymphocytes
lytes	electrolytes

M

M	meter; murmur
Mabs	monoclonal antibodies
MAO	maximal acid output; monoamine oxidase
MAR	multiple antibiotic resistant
MBC	maximal breathing capacity
MBD	minimal brain damage
mc	millicurie
mcg µg	microgram
MCH	mean corpuscular hemoglobin
MCHC	mean corpuscular hemoglobin concentration
MCT	mean circulation time
MCV	mean corpuscular volume
MD	macular degeneration; medical doctor; muscular dystrophy
MDR-TB	multidrug-resistant tuberculosis
MDS	myelodysplastic syndrome
ME	middle ear
MED	minimal effective dose; minimal erythema dose
mEq	milliequivalent
mets	metastasis
M & F	mother and father
MFT	muscle function test
mg	milligram
MG	myasthenia gravis
mgm	milligram
MH	malignant hyperpyrexia; malignant hyperthermia; marital history
MHA	microhemagglutination
MHC	major histocompatibility complex
MI	mitral insufficiency; myocardial infarction
MICU	medical intensive care unit; mobile intensive care unit

MID	multi-infarct dementia
MIDCAB	minimally invasive direct coronary artery bypass
MIP	maximal inspiratory pressure
ml, mL	milliliter
MLD	median lethal dose
mm	millimeter
mm Hg	millimeters of mercury
MM	multiple myeloma; malignant melanoma
MND	motor neuron disease
MNT	medical nutrition therapy
MODY	maturity-onset diabetes of the young
MOM	milk of magnesia
mono	monocytes
MP	metacarpal-phalangeal
MPD	myofacial pain dysfunction
MPJ	metacarpophalangeal joint
MR	mental retardation; metabolic rate; mitral regurgitation
MRD	medical record department
MRI	magnetic resonance imaging
MS	mitral stenosis; multiple sclerosis; musculoskeletal
MSH	melanocyte-stimulating hormone
MSL	midsternal line
MT	medical technician; medical technologist
MTD	right eardrum
MTS	left eardrum
MTX	methotrexate
multip	multipara; multiparous
MV	mitral valve
MVP	mitral valve prolapse
MVPS	Medicare volume performance standard
MY	myopia
myel	myelogram
myop	myopia

N

N	nitrogen
N/C	no complaints
NA	not applicable; numerical aperture
Na	sodium
NaCl	sodium chloride
NAD	no acute disease; no apparent distress
NB	newborn
NBT	nitroblue tetrazolium
NCV	nerve conduction velocity
NED	no evidence of disease
NEG, neg	negative
neuro	neurology
NF	National Formulary; neurofibromatosis
N/G	nasogastric (tube)

ng	*Neisseria gonorrhoeae*
NGU	nongonococcal urethritis
NHL	non-Hodgkin's lymphoma
NICU	neurologic intensive care unit
NIDDM	non–insulin-dependent diabetes mellitus
NK	natural killer (cell)
NKA	no known allergies
NLP	neurolinguistic programming
NM	neuromuscular; nuclear medicine
N & M	nerves and muscles; night and morning
NMR	nuclear magnetic resonance
No.	number
noc, noct	night
NOFTT	nonorganic failure to thrive
NPC	no point of convergence
NPH	neutral protamine Hagedorn
NPN	nonprotein nitrogen
NPO	nothing by mouth
NR	no response
NREM	no rapid eye movements
N/S	normal saline
NS	nephrotic syndrome; normal saline; not stated; not sufficient
NSAID	nonsteroidal anti-inflammatory drug
NSR	normal sinus rhythm
NSU	nonspecific urethritis
Nt	neutralization
N & T	nose and throat
NTD	neural tube defect
NTG	nitroglycerin
N & V	nausea and vomiting
NVA	near visual acuity
NVD	nausea, vomiting, and diarrhea; neck vein distention
NVS	neural vital signs
NYD	not yet diagnosed

O

OA	osteoarthritis
OB	obstetrics
OB-GYN	obstetrics and gynecology
obl	oblique
OBS	organic brain syndrome
Obs	obstetrics
OC	office call; oral contraceptive
OCC	occasional
OCD	obsessive compulsive disorder; oral cholecystogram
OCT	oral contraceptive therapy
OD	overdose; right eye (oculus dexter)
od	once a day

OGN	obstetric-gynecologic-neonatal
OGTT	oral glucose tolerance test
oint	ointment
OJD	osteoarthritic joint disease
OM	otitis media
OME	otitis media with effusion
OMR	optic mark recognition
OOB	out of bed
O & P	ova and parasites
OP	outpatient
OPD	outpatient department
OPG	oculoplethysmography
Ophth	ophthalmic
OPT	outpatient
OPV	oral poliovirus vaccine
OR	operating room
ORIF	open reduction internal fixation
ORT	oral rehydration therapy
Orth	orthopedics
OS	left eye (oculus sinister)
os	mouth
OSA	obstructive sleep apnea
OT	occupational therapy; old tuberculin
OTC	over-the-counter
Oto	otology
OU	each eye (oculus unitas)
oz	ounce
OXT	oxytocin

P

P, $\bar{p}$	after; phosphorus; pulse
P & A	percussion and auscultation
PA	pernicious anemia; physician's assistant; posteroanterior; posterior-anterior; pulmonary artery
PABA	para-aminobenzoic acid
PAC	premature atrial contraction
PACAB	port-access coronary artery bypass
PADP	pulmonary artery diastolic pressure
PALS	pediatric advanced life support
PAMP	pulmonary arterial mean pressure
Pap	Papanicolaou smear
PAR	perennial allergic rhinitis; postanesthetic recovery
PARA (P_1)	full-term infants delivered
paren	parenterally
PASP	pulmonary artery systolic pressure
PAT	paroxysmal atrial tachycardia
Path	pathology
PBC	primary biliary cirrhosis
PBI	protein-bound iodine

PBP	progressive bulbar palsy
PBT_4	protein-bound thyroxine
pc	after meals
PCO, PCOS	polycystic ovary syndrome
PCP	*Pneumocystis carinii* pneumonia
PCT	plasmacrit time
PCU	progressive care unit
PCV	packed cell volume
PD	interpupillary distance; Parkinson's disease; peritoneal dialysis
PDA	patent ductus arteriosus
PDD	pervasive developmental disorder
PDL	periodontal ligament
PE	physical examination
PEA	pulseless electrical activity
Peds	pediatrics
PEEP	positive end-expiratory pressure
PEF	peak expiratory flow rate
PEG	pneumoencephalogram; pneumoencephalography
PEL	permissible exposure limit
per	by; through
PERLA	pupils equally reactive to light and accommodation
PERRLA	pupils equal, round, react to light and accommodation
PET	positron emission tomography; preeclamptic toxemia
PE tube	ventilating tube for the eardrum
PFT	pulmonary function test
PG	pregnant; prostaglandin
PG, 2-h	post-load glucose (number indicates elapsed time)
PGH	pituitary growth hormone
PGL	persistent generalized lymphadenopathy
pH	acidity; hydrogen ion concentration
PH	past history; personal history; public health
PHN	postherpetic neuralgia
PI	present illness
PICU	pulmonary intensive care unit
PID	pelvic inflammatory disease
PIF	peak inspiratory flow
PIP	proximal interphalangeal
PK	pyruvate kinase; pyruvate kinase deficiency
PKR	partial knee replacement
PKU	phenylketonuria
PL	light perception
PLC	platelet count
PLMS	periodic limb movements in sleep
PLS	primary lateral sclerosis
PLTS	platelets
PM	evening or afternoon; physical medicine; polymyositis; postmortem
PMA	progressive muscular atrophy
PMH	past medical history

PMI	point of maximal impulse
PMN	polymorphonuclear neutrophils
PMP	past menstrual period; previous menstrual period
PMR	physical medicine and rehabilitation; polymyalgia rheumatica
PMS	premenstrual syndrome
PMT	premenstrual tension
PMVS	prolapsed mitral valve syndrome
PND	paroxysmal nocturnal dyspnea; postnasal drip
PNH	paroxysmal nocturnal hemoglobinuria
PNS	parasympathetic nervous system; peripheral nervous system
PO, p.o.	by mouth; orally; phone order; postoperative
POC	products of conception
polys	polymorphonuclear leukocytes
POMR	problem-oriented medical record
pos	positive
POS	polycystic ovary syndrome
post-op	postoperatively
PP	postpartum; postprandial (after meals); pulse pressure
PPA pos	phenylpyruvic acid positive
PPBS	postprandial blood sugar
PPD	purified protein derivative
PPLO	pleuropneumonia-like organisms
PPS	postperfusion syndrome; postpolio syndrome
PPV	positive-pressure ventilation
PR	peripheral resistance; pulse rate
pr	by rectum
PRA	plasma renin activity
PRBC	packed red blood cells
PRC	packed red cells
PRE	progressive restrictive exercise
preg	pregnant
preop	preoperative
prep	prepare
primip	primipara; primiparous
PRK	photoreactive keratectomy
prn	as needed
proct	proctology
prog	prognosis
PROM	passive range of motion; premature rupture of membranes
pro time	prothrombin time
PRRE	pupils round, regular, and equal
PSA	prostate-specific antigen
PSP	phenolsulfonphthalein
PSS	progressive systemic sclerosis; physiologic saline solution
psych	psychiatry
PT	paroxysmal tachycardia; physical therapy; prothrombin time

pt	patient; pint
PTA	percutaneous transluminal angioplasty; plasma thromboplastin antecedent, factor XI
PPT	partial prothrombin time
PTB	patellar tendon bearing
PTC	percutaneous transhepatic cholangiography; plasma thromboplastic component; factor XI
PTCA	percutaneous transluminal coronary angioplasty
PTD	permanent and total disability
PTE	parathyroid extract
PTH	parathyroid hormone; parathormone
PTSD	posttraumatic stress disorder
PTT	partial thromboplastin time; prothrombin time
PU	peptic ulcer; pregnancy urine; prostatic urethra
PUD	peptic ulcer disease; pulmonary disease
pul	pulmonary
PV	peripheral vascular; plasma volume; polycythemia vera
P & V	pyloroplasty and vagotomy
PVC	premature ventricular contraction
PVD	peripheral vascular disease
PVE	prosthetic valve endocarditis
PVOD	peripheral vascular occlusive disease
PVS	persistent vegetative state
PVT	paroxysmal ventricular tachycardia
pvt	private
PWB	partial weight-bearing
PWP	pulmonary wedge pressure
Px	prognosis

Q

q	every
qd, q.d.	every day
qh, q.h.	every hour
q 2 h	every 2 hours
QID, qid, q.i.d.	four times a day
qm	every morning
qn	every night
qns	quantity not sufficient
qod	every other day
qoh	every other hour
QOL	quality of life
qs	quantity sufficient
qt	quart; quiet
q.q.	each
quad	quadrant

R

R	rectal; respiration; right
RA	refractory anemia; rheumatoid arthritis; right arm; right atrium

Ra	radium
rad	radiation absorbed dose
RAF	rheumatoid arthritis factor
RAI	radioactive iodine
RAIU	radioactive iodine uptake determination
RAS	reticular activating system
RAST	radioallergosorbent
RAT	radiation therapy
RBBB	right bundle branch block
RBC	red blood cell; red blood count
RBCV	red blood cell volume
RBE	relative biologic effects
RCA	right coronary artery
RD	respiratory distress; retinal detachment
RDA	recommended daily allowance
RDS	respiratory distress syndrome
reg	regular
rehab	rehabilitation
rem	roentgen-equivalent-man
REM	rapid eye movement
RER	renal excretion rate
RES	reticuloendothelial system
RBRVS	resource-based relative value scale
resp	respirations
RF	renal failure; rheumatoid factor; rheumatic fever
RFS	renal function study
RH	right hand
Rh neg	Rhesus factor negative
Rh pos	Rhesus factor positive
RHD	rheumatic heart disease
RIA	radioimmunoassay
RICE	rest, ice, compression, elevate
RIF	right iliac fossa
RIST	radioimmunosorbent
RK	radial keratotomy
RL	right leg
RLC	residual lung capacity
RLD	related living donor
RLE	right lower extremity
RLL	right lower lobe
RLQ	right lower quadrant
RLS	restless legs syndrome
RM	respiratory movement
RML	right mediolateral
RMSF	Rocky Mountain spotted fever
RNA	ribonucleic acid
RND	radical neck dissection
R/O	rule out
ROA	right occipitis anterior
ROM	range of motion; rupture of membranes
ROP	right occipitis posterior

ROPS	roll over protection structures
ROS	review of systems
ROT	right occipitis transverse
RP	relapsing polychondritis; retrograde pyelogram
RPCF	Reiter protein complement fixation
RPF	renal plasma flow
RPG	retrograde pyelogram
rpm	revolutions per minute
RPO	right posterior oblique
RPR	rapid plasma reagin
RQ	respiratory quotient
R & R	rate and rhythm
RR	recovery room; respiratory rate
RSD	reflex sympathetic dystrophy
RSHF	right-sided heart failure
RSI	repetitive stress injuries
RSR	regular sinus rhythm
RSV	right subclavian vein
rt	right; routine
RT	radiation therapy; respiratory therapy
RTA	renal tubular acidosis
rt lat	right lateral
rtd	retarded
RUL	right upper lobe
RU	roentgen unit; routine urinalysis
RUE	right upper extremity
RUL	right upper lobe
RUQ	right upper quadrant
RV	residual volume; right ventricle
RVG	radionuclide ventriculogram
RVH	right ventricular hypertrophy
RVS	relative value schedule
RW	ragweed
Rx	prescription; take; therapy; treatment

S

$\bar{s}$	without
S-A	sinoatrial node
S & A	sugar and acetone
SA	salicylic acid; sinoatrial; sperm analysis; surgeon's assistant
SAAT	serum aspartate aminotransferase
SAB	spontaneous abortion
SACH	solid ankle cushion heel
SACP	serum acid phosphatase
SAD	seasonal affective disorder
SAFP	serum alpha-fetoprotein
SALD	serum aldolase
SAL	sensorineural activity level; sterility assurance level; suction-assisted lipectomy

SALP	salpingectomy; salpingography; serum alkaline phosphatase
Salpx	salpingectomy
SAM	self-administered medication program
SAS	short arm splint; sleep apnea syndrome; social adjustment scale; subarachnoid space
SB	stillbirth
SBE	subacute bacterial endocarditis
SBO	small bowel obstruction
sc, SC	subcutaneous
SC	spinal cord
SCA	sickle cell anemia
SCC	squamous cell carcinoma
SCD	sudden cardiac death
SCI	spinal cord injury
schiz	schizophrenia
SCID	severe combined immune deficiency
SCPK	serum creatine phosphokinase
SCT	sickle cell trait
SD	septal defect; shoulder disarticulation; spontaneous delivery; sudden death
SDAT	senile dementia of Alzheimer's type
SDM	standard deviation of the mean
SDS	sudden death syndrome
sec, s	second
SED	suberythema dose
sed rate	sedimentation rate
seg	segmented neutrophils
SEM	scanning electron microscopy
semi	half
seq	sequela; sequestrum
SES	subcutaneous electric stimulation
sev	sever; severed
SF	scarlet fever; spinal fluid
SG	serum globulin; skin graft
SGA	small for gestational age
s̄ gl	without correction; without glasses
SGGTP	serum gamma-glutamyl transpeptidase
SGOT	serum glutamic oxaloacetic transaminase
SGPT	serum glutamic pyruvic transaminase
SH	serum hepatitis; sex hormone; social history
sh	shoulder
SI	saturation index
SICU	surgical intensive care unit
SIDS	sudden infant death syndrome
SIRS	systemic inflammatory response syndrome
SIS	saline infusion sonohysterography
SISI	short increment sensitivity index
SLAP	serum leucine aminopeptidase
SLE	St. Louis encephalitis; systemic lupus erythematosus
SLPS	serum lipase

SM	simple mastectomy
sm	small
SMA	sequential multiple analysis
SMAC	sequential multiple analysis computer
SMG	senile macular degeneration
SMR	submucous resection
SMRR	submucous resection and rhinoplasty
SNR	signal-to-noise ratio
SNS	sympathetic nervous system; sensory nervous system
SO	salpingo-oophorectomy
SOAP	symptoms, observations, assessments, plan; subjective, objective, assessment, plan
SOB	shortness of breath
SOM	serous otitis media
SONO	sonography
SOP	standard operating procedure
sos	if necessary
SPBI	serum protein-bound iodine
SPE	serum protein electrophoresis
spec	specimen
SPECT	single photon emission computed tomography
SPF	skin protective factor
sp gr	specific gravity
SPHI	serum phosphohexoisomerase
SPK	serum pyruvate kinase
SPP	suprapubic prostatectomy
SPR	scanned projection radiography
SQ	subcutaneous
SR	sedimentation rate; stimulus response; system review
Sr	strontium
SRS	smoker's respiratory syndrome
$\overline{ss}$	half
SS	Signs and symptoms; Sjögren's syndrome; soap solution
SSE	soap suds enema
SSRI	selective serotonin reuptake inhibitor
SSU	sterile supply unit
staph	staphylococcus
stat	immediately
STD	sexually transmitted disease; skin test dose
STH	somatotropic hormone
STK	streptokinase
strep	streptococcus
STS	serologic test for syphilis
STSG	split-thickness skin graft
subcu	subcutaneous
sub-Q	subcutaneous
SUI	stress urinary incontinence
supp	suppository
surg	surgical; surgery
SVC	superior vena cava

SVD	spontaneous vaginal delivery
SVG	saphenous vein graft
SVN	small volume nebulizer
Sx	symptoms

T

T	temperature
T_1–T_{12}	thoracic vertebrae
T_3	triiodothyronine
T_4	thyroxine
TA	therapeutic abortion
T & A	tonsillectomy and adenoidectomy
TAB	therapeutic abortion
tab	tablet
TACT	target air-enema computed tomography
TAF	tumor angiogenesis factor
TAH	total abdominal hysterectomy
TAO	thromboangiitis obliterans
TB	tuberculosis
TBD	total body density
TBF	total body fat
TBG	thyroxine-binding globulin
TBI	thyroxine-binding index
TBW	total body weight
Tc	technetium
TCDB	turn, cough, deep breathe
TCP	time care profile
TD	total disability
TDM	therapeutic drug monitoring
TDT	tone decay test
TEE	transesophageal echocardiography
temp	temperature
TEN	toxic epidermal necrolysis
TENS	transcutaneous electrical nerve stimulation
TES	treadmill exercise score
TF	tactile fremitus
TFS	thyroid function studies
TGA	transposition of great arteries
THR	total hip replacement
TIA	transient ischemic attack
TIA-IR	transient ischemic attack incomplete recovery
TIBC	total iron-binding capacity
TID, tid, t.i.d.	times interval difference; three times a day
tinct	tincture
TKO	to keep open
TKR	total knee replacement
TLC	tender loving care; total lung capacity
TLE	temporal lobe epilepsy
TM	temporomandibular; tympanic membrane
TMD	temporomandibular disease; temporomandibular disorder

TMJ	temporomandibular joint
TMs	tympanic membranes
Tn	normal intraocular tension
TND	term normal delivery
TNF	tumor necrosis factor
TNI	total nodal irradiation
TNM	tumor, nodes, metastases
TO	telephone order
top	topically
TP	testosterone propionate; total protein
TPA	tissue plasminogen activator; *Treponema pallidum* agglutination
TPBF	total pulmonary blood flow
TPI	*Treponema pallidum* immobilization
TPN	total parenteral nutrition
TPR	temperature, pulse, respiration
TPUR	transperineal urethral resection
tr	tincture
TR	tuberculin residue
trach	tracheostomy
TRBF	total renal blood flow
TRH	thyrotropin-releasing hormone
TS	Tourette syndrome
TSD	Tay-Sachs disease
TSE	testicular self-examination
TSH	thyroid-stimulating hormone
TSP	total serum protein
TSS	toxic shock syndrome
TST	tuberculin skin test
TT	thrombin time
TTH	thyrotropic hormone
TULIP	transurethral ultrasound-guided laser-induced proctectomy
TUMT	transurethral microwave therapy
TUR	transurethral resection
TURP	transurethral resection of prostate; prostatectomy
TV	tidal volume; tricuspid valve
TVH	total vaginal hysterectomy
TW	tap water
TWE	tap water enema
Tx	traction; treatment

U

U	units
UA	urinalysis
UAO	upper airway obstruction
UC	ulcerative colitis; urine culture; uterine contractions
UCD	usual childhood diseases
UCG	urinary chorionic gonadotropin; uterine chorionic gonadotropin

UCR	unconditioned reflex
UE	upper extremity
UFR	uroflowmeter; uroflowmetry
UG	upper gastrointestinal; urogenital
UGI	upper gastrointestinal
UK	unknown
UL	upper lobe
ULQ	upper left quadrant
umb	umbilicus
UN	urea nitrogen
ung	ointment
UOQ	upper outer quadrant
UP	uroporphyrin
UPP	urethral pressure profile
UR	upper respiratory
URD	upper respiratory disease
URI	upper respiratory infection
urol	urology
URQ	upper right quadrant
US	ultrasonic; ultrasonography
USP	United States Pharmacopeia
UTI	urinary tract infection
UV	ultraviolet
UVJ	ureterovesical junction

V

VA	vacuum aspiration; visual acuity
vag	vaginal
VB	viable birth
VBAC	vaginal birth after cesarean
VBP	ventricular premature beat
VC	acuity of color vision; vena cava; vital capacity
VCG	vectorcardiogram
VCUG	voiding cystourethrogram
VD	venereal disease
VDG	venereal disease, gonorrhea
VDH	valvular disease of heart
VDRL	Venereal Disease Research Laboratory
VDS	venereal disease, syphilis
VE	visual efficiency
VEP	visual evoked potential
VER	visual evoked response
VF	visual field; vocal fremitus
V fib	ventricular fibrillation
VG	ventricular gallop
VH	vaginal hysterectomy
VHD	valvular heart disease; ventricular heart disease
VI	volume index
vit cap	vital capacity
VLDL	very-low-density lipoprotein

VP	venipuncture; venous pressure
V & P	vagotomy and pyloroplasty
VPC	ventricular premature contraction
VPRC	volume of packed red cells
VS, vs	vital signs
VSD	ventricular septal defect
VTAs	vascular targeting agents
VZV	varicella-zoster virus (chickenpox)

W

W	water
WA	while awake
WB	weight-bearing; whole blood
WBC	white blood cell; white blood count
W/C, w/c	wheelchair
wd	wound
WD, w/d	well-developed
WDWN	well-developed well-nourished
wf	white female
w/n	well-nourished
WNL	within normal limits
w/o	without
WR	Wassermann reaction
wt	weight
w/v	weight by volume

X

x	multiplied by; times
XDP	xeroderma pigmentosum
XM	cross-match
XR	x-ray
XT	exotropia
XU	excretory urogram

Y

y/o	year(s) old
YOB	year of birth
yr, y	year

Z

Z	atomic number; no effect; zero

SECTION 4

Conversions

■ ■ ■

24-HOUR CLOCK (MILITARY TIME) CONVERSION CHART

Time	24-Hour Time	Time	24-Hour Time
12:01 AM	0001	12:01 PM	1201
12:05 AM	0005	12:05 PM	1205
12:30 AM	0030	12:30 PM	1230
12:45 AM	0045	12:45 PM	1245
1:00 AM	0100	1:00 PM	1300
2:00 AM	0200	2:00 PM	1400
3:00 AM	0300	3:00 PM	1500
4:00 AM	0400	4:00 PM	1600
5:00 AM	0500	5:00 PM	1700
6:00 AM	0600	6:00 PM	1800
7:00 AM	0700	7:00 PM	1900
8:00 AM	0800	8:00 PM	2000
9:00 AM	0900	9:00 PM	2100
10:00 AM	1000	10:00 PM	2200
11:00 AM	1100	11:00 PM	2300
12:00 NOON	1200	12:00 MIDNIGHT	2400

TEMPERATURE CONVERSIONS

Fahrenheit–Celsius (Centigrade) Equivalents

F°	C°	F°	C°	F°	C°
32	0	102	38.9	116	46.7
70	21.1	103	39.4	117	47.2
75	23.9	104	40	118	47.8
80	26.7	105	40.6	119	48.3
85	29.4	106	41.1	120	48.9
90	32.2	107	41.7	125	51.7
95	35	108	42.2	130	54.4
96	35.6	109	42.8	135	57.2
97	36.1	110	43.3	140	60
98	36.7	111	43.9	150	65.6
98.6	37	112	44.4	212	100
99	37.2	113	45		
100	37.8	114	45.6		
101	38.3	115	46.1		

To convert Fahrenheit to Celsius, subtract 32 from the Fahrenheit degrees and multiply by 5/9: $C = (F-32) \times 5/9$

Example:
$C = (98.6°F - 32) \times 5/9$
$C = 66.6 \times 5/9$
$C = 333/9$
$C = 37°$
$98.6°F = 37°C$

Example:
$C = (91.4°F - 32) \times 5/9$
$C = 59.4 \times 5/9$
$C = 297/9$
$C = 33°$
$91.4°F = 33°C$

To convert Celsius to Fahrenheit, multiply Celsius degrees by 9/5 and add 32: $F = (C \times 9/5) + 32$

Example:
$F = (37°C \times 9/5) + 32$
$F = (333/5) + 32$
$F = 66.6 + 32$
$F = 98.6°$
$37°C = 98.6°F$

Example:
$F = (38°C \times 9/5) + 32$
$F = (342/5) + 32$
$F = 68.4 + 32$
$F = 100.4°$
$38°C = 100.4°F$

MEASUREMENT EQUIVALENTS AND CONVERSIONS

Metric Equivalents

1 L = 1000 mL
1 L = 1000 cc
1 mL = 1 cc
1 g = 1000 mg
1 mg = 1000 mcg
1 kg = 1000 g

Apothecaries' and Household Equivalents

qt i = pt ii (2)
qt i = ℥ 32
pt i = ℥ 16
℥ i = ℈ viii (8)
1 T = 3 t

Approximate Equivalents between Systems

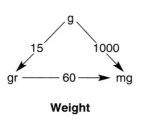

1 g = gr 15
gr i = 60 mg
1 t = 5 mL = 5 cc
℈ i = 4 mL = 4 cc
℥ i = 30 mL = 30 cc
qt i = 1 L = ℥ 32
1 kg = 2.2 lb
1 in = 2.5 cm

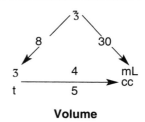

Weight

Volume

Rules for Converting from One System to Another

Volumes

Grains to grams—divide by 15
Drams to cubic centimeters—multiply by 4
Ounces to cubic centimeters—multiply by 30
Minims to cubic millimeters—multiply by 63
Minims to cubic centimeters—multiply by 0.06
Cubic millimeters to minims—divide by 63
Cubic centimeters to minims—multiply by 16
Cubic centimeters to fluid ounces—divide by 30
Liters to pints—divide by 2.1

Weights

Milligrams to grains—multiply by 0.0154
Grams to grains—multiply by 15
Grams to drams—multiply by 0.257
Grams to ounces—multiply by 0.0311

Pounds to kilograms—divide by 2.2
Kilograms to pounds—multiply by 2.2

Lengths

Inches to centimeters—multiply by 2.54
Feet to centimeters—multiply by 30.48
Centimeters to inches—divide by 2.54
Centimeters to feet—divide by 30.48

Converting Measurements

Length	Centimeters	Inches	Feet
1 centimeter	1.000	0.394	0.0328
1 inch	2.54	1.000	0.0833
1 foot	30.48	12.000	1.000
1 yard	91.4	36.00	3.00
1 meter	100.00	39.40	3.28

Volumes	Cubic Centimeters	Fluid Drams	Fluid Ounces	Quarts	Liters
1 cubic centimeter	1.00	0.270	0.033	0.0010	0.0010
1 fluid dram	3.70	1.00	0.125	0.0090	0.0037
1 cubic inch	16.39	4.43	0.554	0.0173	0.0163
1 fluid ounce	29.6	8.00	1.000	0.0312	0.0296
1 quart	946.0	255.0	32.0	1.00	0.946
1 liter	1000.0	270.0	33.80	1.056	1.000

Weights	Grains	Grams	Apothecary Ounces	Pounds
1 grain (gr)	1.000	0.064	0.002	0.0001
1 gram (gm)	15.43	1.000	0.032	0.0022
1 apothecary ounce	480.00	31.1	1.000	0.0685
1 pound	7000.00	454.0	14.58	1.000
1 kilogram	15432.0	1000.0	32.15	2.205

Vital Signs

■ ■ ■

BLOOD PRESSURE

Normal Values

Age 18+	120/80
Age 14–17	120/76
Age 8–13	110/72
Age 2–7	100/64
Age 1 Year	96/64

Factors That Affect Blood Pressure

Factor	Explanation
Gender	Adult males usually have a higher blood pressure than adult females.
Age	As age increases, blood pressure also increases.
Exercise	Physical activity increases blood pressure. Allow patient to rest before taking blood pressure.
Body position	Blood pressure varies according to position of patient. Document position if other than sitting. L. (lying); St. (standing).
Medications	Many medications alter blood pressure.

How High Blood Pressure Is Defined

Category	Systolic/ Diastolic	Recommendations
Stage 1	140–159/90–99	Confirm in 2 months; begin lifestyle modifications
Stage 2	160–179/100–119	Medical evaluation; begin treatment within 1 month
Stage 3	180–209/110–119	Medical evaluation; begin treatment within 1 week
Stage 4	210/120 and over	Immediate medical evaluation and treatment

PULSE

Normal Values

Age 13–Adult	60–100/min
Age 6–12	75–110/min
Age 2–6	75–120/min
Age 1–2	80–130/min
1 mo–1 yr	80–140/min
NB–1 mo	120–160/min

Factors That Affect Pulse

Gender—Females usually have a higher pulse rate than males.
Age—As age increases, pulse rate decreases.
Medications—Stimulants increase pulse rate; depressants decrease pulse rate.
Exercise—Physical activity causes pulse rate to rise.
Metabolism—Anything that affects metabolism also affects pulse rate, such as fever, pregnancy, and so on.

RESPIRATION

Normal Values

Age 16–Adulthood	16–20/min
Age 10–16	17–22/min
Age 1–2	20–40 min
Infant	30–50/min

Factors That Affect Respiration Rate

Age—As age increases, respiration decreases.
Illness—Fever can cause respiration rate to rise.
Drugs—Drugs can alter respiration rate.
Exercise—Exercise increases respiration rate.
Emotions—Emotions can alter respiration (usually increase the rate).

Breath Sounds

Wheezing—Continuous high-pitched sounds. Patient really struggles for breath.
Crackles or Rales—Intermittent sounds that can be wet or dry and vary in pitch. (Need stethoscope.)
Stertor—Sounds like the patient is snoring upon respiration.
Stridor—High-pitched crowing sound, heard during inspiration. Common in croup.
Gurgles—Constant low-pitched wheezing, especially during exhalation. (Need stethoscope.)

TEMPERATURE

Route	Location	Average Range	Thermometer Type
Oral	Covered thermometer should be placed under tongue and off to the side of frenulum linguae.	97.6°F–99.6°F (37°C)	Digital Paper Electronic Follow manufacturer's instructions.
Axillary	Place directly under armpit, centered in the midline.	96.6°F–98.6°F (A) (37.6°C)	Digital Paper Electronic Follow manufacturer's instructions.
Rectal	**Infants:** Insert covered thermometer about ½″ into anal canal **Children:** Insert covered thermometer about 1″ into anal canal **Adults:** Insert covered thermometer about 1½″ into anal canal.	98.6°F–100.6°F (R) (36.4°C)	Digital Electronic Follow manufacturer's instructions.
Aural or Tympanic	Place covered probe into ear canal, sealing the opening.	97.6°F–99.6°F (T) (37°C)	

Factors That Influence Temperature

Time of Day—Lowest in the morning.

Age—The younger the patient, the lower the body temperature.

Patient's Normal Temperature—Always review the chart to see what the patient normally runs.

Environment—The cooler the room, the lower the body temperature.

Pregnancy—Usually higher during pregnancy because of increased metabolism.

Strong Emotions—When a patient is upset, body temperature rises.

Temperature-Pulse-Respiration Ratio

Respiration	Pulse	Temperature (F°)
18	80	99
19 (plus)	88	100
21	96	101
23	104	102
25 (minus)	112	103
27	120	104
28 (minus)	128	105
30	136	106

SECTION 6

Communication Techniques

■ ■ ■

THERAPEUTIC INTERACTION

The Terminally Ill Client

- Most terminal illnesses are accompanied by gradual losses in strength, endurance, mobility, and sensation. Helping the client and family adjust to these losses is important.
- Support for the client and family are the major objectives of care in dealing with the terminally ill client.
- The health professional may need emotional support as well because he or she will lose a valued client relationship, too.
- Communicating with the terminally ill client may be difficult because the process of dying is psychologically and physically stressful for the client and loved ones.
- Common fears include the fear of isolation, pain, dependence, and death itself.
- Be willing to listen if the client expresses the need for discussion.
- The terminally ill client will likely experience some or all of the stages of dying.

The Angry Client

- Anger and hostility are often caused by the medical condition. The goal is to calm the client and to contain the situation.
- Clients who lose much autonomy are prone to anger. Anger that is poorly managed may result in aggression.
- Do not get caught in the circle of anger, but remain calm, objective, firm, and direct.
- Never give in to unreasonable demands; however, public displays of anger in front of other clients should be extinguished without further inciting the client. The following is recommended:
  1. Do not get upset. Do not take the client's anger personally.
  2. Do not interrupt an irrational line of reasoning; just listen.
  3. Keep your tone calm and in control.
  4. If the client is loud and disruptive, lead the client to a quiet and private area to discuss the problem.

5. Mirror the client's statements of anger to exhibit your understanding of the problem.
6. If the client refuses to calm down, ask him or her to wait a few moments alone in an exam room. This may have a calming effect; however, allowing the patient to wait too long may have the opposite effect.
7. A psychiatric consultation may be indicated.

The Sensory-Impaired Client

■ For hearing-impaired and foreign-language-speaking clients, an interpreter may be necessary; otherwise, position yourself directly in front of the client and speak slowly.
■ For the sight impaired, ask the client, "How can I be of assistance?" rather than taking the client's hand or arm and directing her.
■ When communicating with sensory-impaired clients, be open, flexible, and supportive.

Children

Most people must make an effort to adjust to being ill, but this can be more problematic for children, who may not understand their situation and may even feel that illness is a means of punishment.

■ Be aware of your feelings toward children. They can sense how you feel.
■ Establish a friendly relationship with children.
■ Speak to children in quiet, pleasant tones while kneeling down to meet their level.
■ Use language (without clichés) that is appropriate to the child's age.
■ Allow children to choose in situations in which any choice will be correct.
■ Allow children to assist in their treatment without losing control.
■ The longer children have to wait, the more irritable they become.
■ Children tend to regress when ill.
■ Be truthful to children and help them deal with their fears and feelings. Explain what you are going to do and why; do so as close to the time of the procedure as possible.
■ Never shame a child and do not use labels such as baby or sissy.
■ Offer rewards such as stickers, inexpensive toys, and the like.
■ If safe, allow the child to play with equipment to be used.
■ Demonstrate the procedure on a doll.
■ Describe sensations the child may feel during or after the procedure.
■ Do not provide more information than is necessary.
■ Infants should be comforted by being held at each visit and after painful procedures.
■ Developing trust in infants: Three C's—*consistency* of approach, *constancy* of presence, and *continuity* of care.
  1. An infant expresses need through generalized behavior.
  2. The caregiver responds, satisfying the infant's need.
  3. The infant predicts the caregiver's response and repeats the behavior.
  4. The caregiver responds in a consistent manner, satisfying the infant's need.

5. The infant develops trust, and when the need recurs, is confident that the caregiver will respond appropriately.

The Adolescent Client

Adolescents are caught between childhood and adulthood. As a result, they often demand independence, yet require the comfort and consoling frequently afforded children.

■ Permit privacy and the right to be examined in the parent's absence.
■ Be prepared for adolescent clients not having accurate information about sex.
■ Treat adolescents with respect and dignity.
■ Set limits that are fair and consistent.

The Elderly Client

The elderly are presented with myriad problems and challenges associated with aging, ranging from physical disability to social isolation.

■ Allow additional time for tasks we complete easily and quickly.
■ Afford the elderly physical and environmental comforts.
■ As humans are creatures of habit, the elderly find comfort in a routine, so allow for a set schedule.
■ Do not be overattentive or overprotective.
■ Afford the elderly as much independence as possible.

The Frightened Client

■ Denial of fear is a common defense mechanism.
■ Frightened clients are often uncooperative, because to accept help is to acknowledge that the fear exists. This is especially true among male clients.
■ Recognize, accept, and help the client deal with the fear.
■ Afford as much control over the situation as possible.
■ Intense fear can bring about a panic response, causing the person to withdraw. Act for the person.

Abusive and Abused Clients

■ Phases of violence
   1. Triggering: A stressor precipitates verbal aggression or threats.
   2. Escalation: The threat of aggression heightens as the perpetrator becomes more enraged.
   3. Crisis: The perpetrator loses control over anger and resorts to physical aggression.
   4. Recovery: The perpetrator calms down and returns to the pre-triggering state.
   5. Postcrisis: The perpetrator will either rationalize his behavior or attempt to make amends and promise not to be abusive again, or both.
■ Physical injuries should be treated promptly.
■ Resource material should be available to refer clients to agencies skilled in handling such problems.
■ Focus on the victim and provide assurances of self-worth.

■ Observe the abuser's personal space to avoid being perceived as a threat. Accept the abuser's feelings, but not the violent behavior.

Interacting with Significant Others

■ Family and friends form an emotional support group for the client and should not be discounted. Minister to the needs and questions of the client's loved ones.

■ In most cases, the wishes of the client should be addressed regarding visitation of loved ones or who can be given information regarding the client.

■ Young children need to be accompanied by an adult; however, as children approach adolescence, they require more autonomy and privacy.

■ Waiting friends and relatives should be periodically notified of the progress of the client and informed of any delays.

■ Family and friends are an important factor in the client's healing; their concerns can be as important to successful treatment as the client's.

SECTION 7

Dosage Calculations

■ ■ ■

DOSAGE CALCULATION FORMULAS

Dosage: Formula Method

Step 1.   Convert
Step 2.   Think
Step 3.   Calculate: $\dfrac{D}{H} \times Q = X$

Dosage: Ratio-Proportion Method

Step 1.   Convert
Step 2.   Think
Step 3.   Calculate: $\dfrac{\text{Dosage on hand}}{\text{Volume on hand}} = \dfrac{\text{Dosage desired}}{\text{X volume}}$

Dimensional Analysis Method

The problem:

> You are asked to administer 40 mg of furosemide.
> It is packaged 10 mg/mL in an 8 mL ampule.

Set up as:

$$40 \text{ mg} : x \text{ mL} : : 10 \text{ mg} : 1 \text{ mL}$$

Multiply the means. $40 : x : : 10 : 1$

$$x \times 10 = 10x$$

Multiply the extremes. $40 : x : : 10 : 1$

$$40 \times 1 = 40$$

Set up as:

$$10x = 40$$

(continues)

To solve for x, divide both sides by 10.

$$10x \div 10 = 1x \text{ or } x$$
$$40 \div 10 = 4$$

Solution: x = 4 mL
Therefore, administer 4 mL to deliver 40 mg of furosemide.

Intravenous Flow Rate

Total mL/Total h = mL/h

$$\frac{\text{Total mL}}{\text{Total min}} \times 60 \text{ min/h} = \text{mL/h}$$

$$\frac{V \text{ (mL)}}{T \text{ (min)}} \times C \text{ (gtt/mL)} = R \text{ (gtt/min)}$$

Shortcut

IV flow rate: $\dfrac{\text{mL/h}}{\text{Drop factor constant}} = R \text{ (gtt/min)}$

Body Surface Area

Metric: BSA $(m^2) = \sqrt{\dfrac{h + (cm) \times wt \text{ (kg)}}{3600}}$

Household: BSA $(m^2) = \sqrt{\dfrac{h + (in) \times wt \text{ (lb)}}{3131}}$

MEDICATION ADMINISTRATION RIGHTS

Application of Seven Rights

1. Right patient
2. Right drug
3. Right dose
4. Right route
5. Right time
6. Right technique
7. Right documentation

Glossary

■ ■ ■

A

abrasion (ah-**BRAY**-zhun): An injury in which superficial layers of skin are scraped or rubbed away; treatment involving scraping or rubbing away skin.

abruptio placentae (ab-**RUP**-shee-oh plah-**SEN**-tee): An abnormal condition in which the placenta separates from the uterine wall prematurely before the birth of the fetus.

abscess (**AB**-sess): A localized collection of pus within a circumscribed area that is associated with tissue destruction.

Achilles tendinitis (ten-dih-**NIGH**-tis): Inflammation of the Achilles tendon caused by excessive stress being placed on the tendon.

achlorhydria (ah-klor-**HIGH**-dree-ah): The absence of hydrochloric acid from gastric secretions.

acne vulgaris (**ACK**-nee vul-**GAY**-ris): A chronic inflammatory disease that is characterized by pustular eruptions of the skin in or near the sebaceous glands.

acquired immune deficiency syndrome: The advanced stage of HIV infection.

acromegaly (**ack**-roh-**MEG**-ah-lee): Enlargement of the extremities (hands and feet) caused by excessive secretion of the growth hormone *after* puberty.

acrophobia (**ack**-roh-**FOH**-bee-ah): An excessive fear of being in high places.

actinic keratosis (ack-**TIN**-ick **kerr**-ah-**TOH**-sis): A precancerous skin lesion caused by excessive exposure to the sun.

acute nasopharyngitis (**nay**-zoh-**far**-in-**JIGH**-tis): Inflammation of the nose and throat; among the terms used to describe the common cold; also known as an upper respiratory infection.

acute respiratory distress syndrome: A type of lung failure resulting from many different disorders that cause pulmonary edema.

addiction: Compulsive, uncontrollable dependence on a substance, habit, or action to the degree that stopping causes severe emotional, mental, or physiologic reactions.

Addison's disease (**AD**-ih-sonz): A progressive disease in which the adrenal glands do not produce enough cortisol; if untreated, it can produce a life-threatening addisonian crisis.

adenitis (ad-eh-**NIGH**-tis): Inflammation of a gland.

adenocarcinoma (ad-eh-noh-**kar**-sih-**NOH**-mah): Any one of a large group of carcinomas derived from glandular tissue.

adenoma (ad-eh-**NOH**-mah): A benign tumor in which the cells form recognizable glandular structures.

adenoma, pituitary (ad-eh-**NOH**-mah): A benign tumor of the pituitary gland that causes excess hormone secretion. An ACTH-secreting tumor stimulates the excess production of cortisol that causes most cases of Cushing's syndrome.

adenoma, prolactin-producing: A benign tumor of the pituitary gland that causes it to produce too much prolactin; also known as a prolactinoma.

adenomalacia (ad-eh-noh-mah-**LAY**-shee-ah): Abnormal softening of a gland.

adenosclerosis (ad-eh-noh-skleh-**ROH**-sis): Abnormal hardening of a gland.

adenosis (ad-eh-**NOH**-sis): Any disease condition of a gland.

adhesion (ad-**HEE**-zhun): A band of fibrous tissue that holds structures together abnormally.

adrenalitis (ah-**dree**-nal-**EYE**-tis): Inflammation of the adrenal glands.

adrenitis (ad-reh-**NIGH**-tis): Inflammation of the adrenal glands.

adrenomegaly (ah-**dree**-noh-**MEG**-ah-lee): Enlargement of the adrenal glands.

adrenopathy (ad-ren-**OP**-ah-thee): Any disease of the adrenal glands.

aerophagia (ay-er-oh-**FAY**-jee-ah): The spasmodic swallowing of air followed by eructations.

agoraphobia (ag-oh-rah-**FOH**-bee-ah): An overwhelming and irrational fear of leaving the familiar setting of home or venturing into the open.

albinism (**AL**-bih-niz-um): An inherited deficiency or absence of pigment in the skin, hair, and eyes due to an abnormality in production of melanin.

albuminuria (al-byou-mih-**NEW**-ree-ah): The presence of the serum protein albumin in the urine.

alcoholism (**AL**-koh-hol-izm): Chronic dependence or abuse of alcohol with specific signs and symptoms of withdrawal.

aldosteronism (al-**DOSS**-teh-roh-**niz**-em or al-doh-**STER**-ohn-izm): An abnormality of electrolyte balance caused by excessive secretion of aldosterone.

allergic rhinitis (rye-**NIGH**-tis), commonly referred to as an **allergy**, is an allergic reaction to airborne allergens that causes an increased flow of mucus.

allergy: An overreaction by the body to a particular antigen; also known as hypersensitivity.

alopecia (al-oh-**PEE**-shee-ah): The partial or complete loss of hair; also known as baldness.

alopecia areata: A disease of unknown cause in which there are well-defined bald areas, usually on the scalp and face.

alopecia capitis totalis: A condition characterized by the loss of all the hair on the scalp.

alopecia universalis: The total loss of hair on all parts of the body.

Alzheimer's disease (ALTZ-high-merz): A group of disorders associated with degenerative changes in the brain structure leading to characteristic symptoms that included progressive memory loss, impaired cognition, and personality changes.

amblyopia (am-blee-**OH**-pee-ah): Dimness of vision or the partial loss of sight without detectable disease of the eye.

amebic dysentery (ah-**MEE**-bik **DIS**-en-**ter**-ee): An intestinal infection caused by *Entamoeba histolytica amoeba.*

amenorrhea (ah-**men**-oh-**REE**-ah *or* ay-**men**-oh-**REE**-ah): The absence of menstrual periods. This condition is normal only before puberty, during pregnancy, while breast-feeding, and after menopause.

ametropia (am-eh-**TROH**-pee-ah): An error of refraction in which only objects located a finite distance from the eye are focused on the retina.

amnesia (am-**NEE**-zee-ah): A disturbance in the memory marked by total or partial inability to recall past experiences.

amyotrophic lateral sclerosis (ah-**my**-oh-**TROH**-fick): A degenerative disease of the motor neurons in which patients become progressively weaker until they are completely paralyzed; also known as Lou Gehrig's disease.

anaphylaxis (an-ah-fih-**LACK**-sis): A severe response to a foreign substance such as a drug, food, insect venom, or chemical.

anaplasia (an-ah-**PLAY**-zee-ah): Change in the structure of cells and in their orientation to each other.

anemia (ah-**NEE**-mee-ah): A disorder characterized by lower than normal levels of red blood cells in the blood.

anemia, aplastic (ay-**PLAS**-tick ah-**NEE**-mee-ah): A marked absence of *all* formed blood elements.

anemia, Cooley's: A group of genetic disorders characterized by short-lived red blood cells that lack the normal ability to produce hemoglobin; also known as thalassemia.

anemia, hemolytic: A condition in which red blood cells are destroyed faster than the bone marrow can replace them.

anemia, megaloblastic (MEG-ah-loh-**blas**-tick ah-**NEE**-mee-ah): A form of anemia in which the bone marrow produces large abnormal red blood cells with a reduced capacity to carry oxygen.

anemia, pernicious: An autoimmune disorder that results in the inability of the body to absorb vitamin B_{12} normally.

anemia, sickle cell: A genetic disorder that causes abnormal hemoglobin that results in the red blood cells assuming an abnormal sickle shape.

angiitis (an-je-**EYE**-tis): Inflammation of a blood or lymph vessel; also known as vasculitis.

angina pectoris (an-**JIGH**-nah *or* **AN**-jih-nuh **PECK**-toh-riss): Severe episodes of spasmodic choking or suffocating chest pain caused by an insufficient supply of oxygen to the heart muscle.

angiogenesis (an-jee-oh-**JEN**-eh-sis): The ability of a tumor to support its growth by creating its own blood supply.

angiomegaly (an-jee-oh-**MEG**-ah-lee): Abnormal enlargement of blood vessels.

angionecrosis (an-jee-oh-neh-**KROH**-sis): Death of the walls of blood vessels.

angiosclerosis (an-jee-oh-skleh-**ROH**-sis): Abnormal hardening of the walls of blood vessels.

angiospasm (AN-jee-oh-**spazm**): Spasmodic contraction of the blood vessels.

angiostenosis (an-jee-oh-steh-**NOH**-sis): Abnormal narrowing of a blood vessel.

anhidrosis (an-high-**DROH**-sis): The condition of lacking or being without sweat.

anisocoria (an-ih-so-**KOH**-ree-ah): A condition in which the pupils are unequal in size.

ankylosing spondylitis (ang-kih-**LOH**-sing **spon**-dih-**LYE**-tis): Rheumatoid arthritis characterized by progressive stiffening of the spine caused by fusion of the vertebral bodies.

ankylosis (ang-kih-**LOH**-sis): Loss or absence of mobility in a joint due to disease, an injury, or a surgical procedure.

anomaly (ah-**NOM**-ah-lee): A deviation from what is regarded as normal.

anonychia (an-oh-**NICK**-ee-ah): Pertaining to the absence of fingernails or toenails.

anorchism (an-**OR**-kizm): The congenital absence of one or both testicles.

anorexia (an-oh-**RECK**-see-ah): The lack or loss of appetite for food.

anorexia nervosa: An eating disorder characterized by a refusal to maintain a minimally normal body weight and an intense fear of gaining weight.

anovulation (an-ov-you-**LAY**-shun): The failure to ovulate, although menstruation may continue to occur.

anoxia (ah-**NOCK**-see-ah): The absence or almost complete absence of oxygen from inspired gases, arterial blood, or tissues.

anteversion (an-tee-**VER**-zhun): Abnormal tipping, tilting, or turning forward of the entire uterus, including the cervix.

anthracosis (an-thrah-**KOH**-sis): A form of pneumoconiosis caused by coal dust in the lungs; also known as black lung disease.

anuresis (an-you-**REE**-sis): The complete suppression of urine formation by the kidneys; also known as anuria.

anuria (ah-**NEW**-ree-ah): See anuresis.

anxiety state: A feeling of apprehension, tension, or uneasiness that stems from the anticipation of danger, the source of which is largely unknown or unrecognized.

aphakia (ah-**FAY**-kee-ah): The absence of the lens of an eye after cataract extraction.

aphasia (ah-**FAY**-zee-ah): A condition, often due to brain damage associated with a stroke, in which there is the loss of the ability to speak, write, or comprehend speech or the spoken word.

aphonia (ah-**FOH**-nee-ah): Loss of the ability to produce normal speech sounds.

aphthous ulcers (AF-thus): Recurrent blister-like sores that break and form lesions on the soft tissues lining the mouth; also known as canker sores.

aplasia (ah-**PLAY**-zee-ah): Lack of development of an organ or tissue.

apnea (**AP**-nee-ah *or* ap-**NEE**-ah): The absence of spontaneous respiration.

appendicitis (ah-**pen**-dih-**SIGH**-tis): Inflammation of the appendix.

arrhythmia, cardiac (ah-**RITH**-mee-ah): An irregularity or the loss of normal rhythm of the heartbeat; also known as dysrhythmia.

arteriomalacia (ar-**tee**-ree-oh-mah-**LAY**-shee-ah): Abnormal softening of the walls of an artery or arteries.

arterionecrosis (ar-tee-ree-oh-neh-**KROH**-sis): Tissue death of an artery or arteries.

arteriosclerosis (ar-**tee**-ree-oh-skleh-**ROH**-sis): Abnormal hardening of the walls of an artery or arteries.

arteriostenosis (ar-**tee**-ree-oh-steh-**NOH**-sis): Abnormal narrowing of an artery or arteries.

arteritis (**ar**-teh-**RYE**-tis): Inflammation of an artery.

arthralgia (ar-**THRAL**-jee-ah): Pain in a joint or joints.

arthritis (ar-**THRIGH**-tis): Inflammation of one or more joints.

arthritis, gouty: Arthritis associated with the formation of uric acid crystals in the joint as the result of hyperuricemia.

arthritis, juvenile rheumatoid: Arthritis that affects children, with pain and swelling in the joints, skin rash, fever, slowed growth, and fatigue.

arthritis, rheumatoid: Autoimmune disorder in which the synovial membranes are inflamed and thicken.

arthrosclerosis (**ar**-throh-skleh-**ROH**-sis): Stiffness of the joints, especially in the elderly.

asbestosis (**ass**-beh-**STOH**-sis): A form of pneumoconiosis caused by asbestos particles found in the lungs of workers from the ship building and construction trades.

asphyxia (ass-**FICK**-see-ah): Pathologic changes caused by a lack of oxygen in air that is inhaled.

asphyxiation (ass-**fick**-see-**AY**-shun): Any interruption of breathing that results in the loss of consciousness or death; also known as suffocation.

asthma (**AZ**-mah): A chronic allergic disorder characterized by episodes of severe breathing difficulty, coughing, and wheezing.

astigmatism (ah-**STIG**-mah-tizm): A condition in which the eye does not focus properly because of unequal curvatures of the cornea.

ataxia (ah-**TACK**-see-ah): Inability to coordinate the muscles in the execution of voluntary movement.

atelectasis (**at**-ee-**LEK**-tah-sis): A condition in which the lung fails to expand because air cannot pass beyond the bronchioles; also known as a collapsed lung.

atheroma (ath-er-**OH**-mah): Fatty deposit within the wall of an artery.

atherosclerosis (**ath**-er-oh-skleh-**ROH**-sis): Hardening and narrowing of the arteries due to a buildup of cholesterol plaques.

atonic (ah-**TON**-ick): Lack of normal muscle tone.

atrophy (**AT**-roh-fee): Weakness and wasting away.

attention deficit disorder: A condition in which a child has a short attention span and impulsiveness that are inappropriate for the child's developmental age.

attention deficit hyperactivity disorder: A pattern of inattention and hyperactivity that are inappropriate for the child's developmental age.

autistic disorder (aw-**TISS**-tick): A disorder in which a young child cannot develop normal social relationships, behaves in compulsive and ritualistic ways, and frequently has poor communication skills; also known as autism.

autism (**AW**-tizm): See autistic disorder.

autoimmune disorder (**aw**-toh-ih-**MYOUN**): A disorder of the immune system in which the body attacks itself.

azoospermia (ay-**zoh**-oh-**SPER**-mee-ah): The absence of sperm in the semen.

B

bacteriuria (back-**tee**-ree-**YOU**-ree-ah): The presence of bacteria in the urine.

balanitis (**bal**-ah-**NIGH**-tis): Inflammation of the glans penis, usually associated with phimosis.

Becker's muscular dystrophy (**BECK**-urz): A less severe form of muscular dystrophy that does not appear until early adolescence or adulthood.

Bell's palsy: Paralysis of the facial nerve (seventh cranial) that causes drooping only on the affected side of the face.

benign prostatic hypertrophy: An abnormal enlargement of the prostate gland.

bipolar disorder: A clinical course characterized by the occurrence of manic episodes alternating with depressive episodes; also known as manic-depressive disorder.

birthmark: See hemangioma and port-wine stain.

blastoma (blas-**TOH**-mah): A neoplasm composed of immature undifferentiated cells.

blepharedema (**blef**-ahr-eh-**DEE**-mah): Swelling of the eyelid.

blepharitis (**blef**-ah-**RYE**-tis): Inflammation of the eyelid.

blepharoptosis (**blef**-ah-roh-**TOH**-sis *or* blef-ah-rop-**TOH**-sis): Drooping of the upper eyelid.

blindness: The inability to see.

botulism (**BOT**-you-lizm): Food poisoning that is characterized by paralysis and is often fatal, caused by *Clostridium botulinum*.

bradycardia (**brad**-ee-**KAR**-dee-ah): An abnormally slow heartbeat.

bradykinesia (**brad**-ee-kih-**NEE**-zee-ah *or* brad-ee-kih-**NEE**-zhuh): Extreme slowness in movement.

bradypnea (**brad**-ihp-**NEE**-ah *or* brad-ee-**NEE**-ah): An abnormally slow rate of respiration, usually less than 10 breaths per minute.

brain tumor: An abnormal growth within the brain that may be either benign or malignant.

breast augmentation: Mammoplasty to increase breast size.

breech presentation: An abnormal birth position in which the buttocks or feet of the fetus are presented first.

bronchiectasis (brong-kee-**ECK**-tah-sis): Chronic dilation of bronchi or bronchioles resulting from an earlier lung infection that was not cured.

bronchitis (brong-**KYE**-tis): Inflammation of the bronchial walls.

bronchoplegia (brong-koh-**PLEE**-jee-ah): Paralysis of the walls of the bronchi.

bronchopneumonia (brong-koh-new-**MOH**-nee-ah): A form of pneumonia that begins in the bronchioles.

bronchorrhagia (brong-koh-**RAY**-jee-ah): Bleeding from the bronchi.

bronchorrhea (brong-koh-**REE**-ah): An excessive discharge of mucus from the bronchi.

bruit (BREW-ee *or* **BROOT**): An abnormal sound or murmur heard in auscultation.

bruxism (BRUCK-sizm): Involuntary grinding or clenching of the teeth that usually occurs during sleep and is associated with tension or stress.

bulimia (byou-**LIM**-ee-ah *or* boo-**LEE**-mee-ah): An eating disorder characterized by episodes of binge eating followed by self-induced vomiting or misuse of laxatives; also known as bulimia nervosa.

bulla (BULL-ah): A large blister that is *more than* 0.5 cm in diameter.

burn, first-degree: A burn that causes no blisters and only superficial damage to the epidermis; also known as a superficial burn.

burn, second-degree: A burn that causes blisters and superficial damage to the epidermis; also known as a partial thickness burn.

burn, third-degree: A burn that damages the epidermis, corium, and subcutaneous layers; also known as a full-thickness burn.

burn: An injury to body tissues caused by heat, flame, electricity, sun, chemicals, or radiation.

bursitis (ber-**SIGH**-tis): Inflammation of a bursa.

byssinosis (biss-ih-**NOH**-sis): A form of pneumoconiosis caused by cotton, flax, or hemp dust in the lungs; also known as brown lung disease.

C

calciuria (kal-sih-**YOU**-ree-ah): The presence of calcium in the urine.

callus (KAL-us): A thickening of part of the skin on the hands or feet caused by repeated rubbing; the bulging deposit that forms around the area of the break in a fractured bone.

carbuncle (KAR-bung-kul): A cluster of furuncles that result in extensive sloughing of skin and scar formation.

carcinoma (kar-sih-**NOH**-mah): A malignant tumor that occurs in epithelial tissue.

carcinoma, basal cell: A malignant tumor of the basal cell layer of the epidermis.

carcinoma in situ: A malignant tumor in its original position that has not yet disturbed or invaded the surrounding tissues.

cardiorrhexis (kar-dee-oh-**RECK**-sis): Rupture of the heart.

carditis (kar-**DYE**-tis): Inflammation of the heart.

carpal tunnel syndrome (KAR-pul): Inflammation of the tendons passing through the carpal tunnel of the wrist.

cataract (KAT-ah-rakt): Loss of transparency of the lens of the eye.

catatonic (kat-ah-**TON**-ick): Behavior marked by a lack of responsiveness, stupor, and a tendency to remain in a fixed posture.

causalgia (kaw-**ZAL**-jee-ah): Intense burning pain after an injury to a sensory nerve.

cellulitis (sell-you-**LYE**-tis): A diffuse infection of connective tissue with severe inflammation within the layers of the skin.

cephalalgia (sef-ah-**LAL**-jee-ah): Pain in the head; also known as a headache or cephalodynia.

cephalodynia: See cephalalgia.

cerebral palsy (SER-eh-bral *or* seh-**REE**-bral **PAWL**-zee): A condition caused by a brain injury that occurs during pregnancy, birth, or soon after birth that is characterized by poor muscle control and other neurologic deficiencies

cerebrovascular accident (ser-eh-broh-**VAS**-kyou-lar): Damage to the brain when the blood flow to the brain is disrupted because a blood vessel supplying it is blocked; also known as a stroke.

cervical radiculopathy (rah-**dick**-you-**LOP**-ah-thee): Nerve pain caused by pressure on the spinal nerve roots in the neck region.

cervicitis (ser-vih-**SIGH**-tis): Inflammation of the cervix.

chalazion (kah-**LAY**-zee-on): zee-on): A localized swelling of the eyelid resulting from obstruction of one of the oil-producing glands of the eyelid.

Cheyne-Stokes respiration (CHAYN-STOHKS): A pattern of alternating periods of hyperpnea (rapid breathing), hypopnea (slow breathing), and apnea (the absence of breathing).

chickenpox: An acute highly contagious viral disease caused by the herpes virus *Varicella zoster*.

chlamydia (klah-**MID**-ee-ah): A highly contagious sexually transmitted disease caused by the bacterium *Chlamydia trachomatis*.

chloasma (kloh-**AZ**-mah): A pigmentation disorder characterized by brownish spots on the face; also known as melasma or the mask of pregnancy.

cholecystalgia (koh-lee-sis-**TAL**-jee-ah): Pain in the gallbladder.

cholecystitis (koh-lee-sis-**TYE**-tis): Inflammation of the gallbladder.

cholelithiasis (koh-lee-lih-**THIGH**-ah-sis): The presence of gallstones in the gallbladder or bile ducts.

cholera (KOL-er-ah): An intestinal infection caused by *Vibrio cholerae*.

chondritis (kon-**DRY**-tis): Inflammation of cartilage.

chondroma (kon-**DROH**-mah): Benign tumor derived from cartilage cells.

chondromalacia (kon-droh-mah-**LAY**-shee-**ah**): Abnormal softening of the cartilage.

chondropathy (kon-**DROP**-ah-thee): A disease of the cartilage.

chronic obstructive pulmonary disease: A general term used to describe a group of respiratory conditions characterized by chronic airflow limitations.

cicatrix (sick-**AY**-tricks *or* **SICK**-ah-tricks): A "normal" scar resulting from the healing of a wound.

cirrhosis (sih-**ROH**-sis): A progressive degenerative disease of the liver characterized by disturbance of structure and function of the liver.

claustrophobia (**klaws**-troh-**FOH**-bee-ah): An abnormal fear of being in narrow or enclosed spaces.

cleft lip: A congenital defect resulting in a deep fissure of the lip running upward to the nose; also known as a hare lip.

cleft palate: A congenital fissure of the palate that involves the upper lip, hard palate, and/or soft palate.

clubbing: Abnormal curving and shine on the nails that is often accompanied by enlargement of the fingertips. This condition can be hereditary or caused by changes associated with oxygen deficiencies related to coronary or pulmonary disease.

cognition (kog-**NISH**-un): The mental activities associated with thinking, learning, and memory.

colpitis (kol-**PYE**-tis): Inflammation of the lining of the vagina; also known as vaginitis.

coma (**KOH**-mah): A profound state of unconsciousness marked by the absence of spontaneous eye movements, no response to painful stimuli, and no vocalization.

comatose (**KOH**-mah-tohs): The condition of being in a coma.

comedo (**KOM**-eh-doh): A lesion formed by the buildup of sebum and keratin in a hair follicle.

compulsions: Repetitive behaviors the goal of which is to prevent or reduce anxiety or stress.

concussion (kon-**KUSH**-un): A violent shaking up or jarring of the brain.

congenital disorder (kon-**JEN**-ih-tahl): An abnormal condition that exists at the time of birth and may be caused by a developmental disorder before birth, prenatal influences, premature birth, or injuries during birth.

congestive heart failure: A syndrome in which the heart is unable to pump enough blood to meet the body's needs for oxygen and nutrients.

conjunctivitis (kon-**junk**-tih-**VYE**-tis): Inflammation of the conjunctiva; also known as pinkeye.

conscious: State of being awake, aware, and responding appropriately.

constipation: A decrease in frequency in the passage of stools, or difficulty in passing hard, dry stools.

contracture (kon-**TRACK**-chur): Abnormal shortening of muscle tissues making the muscle resistant to stretching.

contusion (kon-**TOO**-zhun): An injury that does not break the skin and is characterized by swelling, discoloration, and pain.

contusion, cerebral: Bruising of brain tissue as a result of a head injury.

convergence (kon-**VER**-jens): The simultaneous inward movement of both eyes in an effort to maintain single binocular vision as an object comes nearer.

conversion disorder: A change in function, such as the paralysis of an arm, that suggests a physical disorder but has no physical cause.

convulsion: A sudden, violent, involuntary contraction of a group of muscles caused by a disturbance in brain function; also known as a seizure.

convulsion, clonic: A state marked by alternate contraction and relaxation of muscles resulting in jerking movements of the face, trunk, or extremities.

convulsion, tonic: A state of continuous muscular contraction that results in rigidity and violent spasms.

corneal abrasion: An injury, such as a scratch or irritation, to the outer layers of the cornea.

corneal ulcer: Pitting of the cornea caused by an infection or injury.

coronary artery disease: Atherosclerosis of the coronary arteries that may cause angina pectoris, myocardial infarction, and sudden death

coronary thrombosis (KOR-uh-**nerr**-ee throm-**BOH**-sis): Damage to the heart caused by a thrombus blocking a coronary artery.

craniocele (**KRAY**-nee-oh-**seel**): A congenital gap in the skull with herniation of brain substance; also known as an encephalocele.

craniomalacia (**kray**-nee-oh-mah-**LAY**-shee-ah): Abnormal softening of the skull.

creatinuria (kree-at-ih-**NEW**-ree-ah): An increased concentration of creatine in the urine.

crepitation (**krep**-ih-**TAY**-shun): Crackling sensation that is felt and heard when the ends of a broken bone move together; also know as crepitus.

crepitus (**KREP**-ih-tus): See crepitation.

cretinism (**CREE**-tin-izm): A congenital lack of thyroid secretion.

Crohn's disease: A chronic autoimmune disorder involving any part of the gastrointestinal tract but most commonly resulting in scarring and thickening of the walls of the ileum, the colon, or both.

croup (**KROOP**): An acute respiratory syndrome in children and infants characterized by obstruction of the larynx, hoarseness, and a barking cough.

crust: A collection of dried serum and cellular debris on the skin.

cryptorchidism (krip-**TOR**-kih-dizm): A developmental defect in which one testis fails to descend into the scrotum; also known as an undescended testis.

Cushing's syndrome (**KUSH**-ingz **SIN**-drohm): A condition caused by prolonged exposure to high levels of cortisol produced by the body or taken as medication.

cyanosis (**sigh**-ah-**NOH**-sis): Blue discoloration of the skin caused by a lack of adequate oxygen.

cyst: A closed sac or pouch containing fluid or semisolid material.

cystalgia (sis-**TAL**-jee-ah): Pain in the urinary bladder.

cystic fibrosis (**SIS**-tick figh-**BROH**-sis): A genetic disorder in which the lungs are clogged with large quantities of abnormally thick mucus and the digestive system is impaired by thick gluelike mucus that interferes with digestive juices.

cystitis (sis-**TYE**-tis): Inflammation of the bladder.

cystocele (**SIS**-toh-seel): A hernia of the bladder through the vaginal wall.

cystodynia (**sis**-toh-**DIN**-ee-ah): Pain in the urinary bladder.

cystolith (**SIS**-toh-lith): Presence of stones in the urinary bladder.

cystoptosis (**sis**-top-**TOH**-sis *or* **sis**-toh-**TOH**-sis): Prolapse of the bladder into the urethra.

cystorrhagia (**sis**-toh-**RAY**-jee-ah): Bleeding from the bladder.

cystorrhexis (**sis**-toh-**RECK**-sis): Rupture of the bladder.

cytomegalovirus (**sigh**-toh-**meg**-ah-loh-**VYE**-rus): An infection caused by a group of large herpes-type viruses with a wide variety of disease effects.

D

dacryocystitis (**dack**-ree-oh-sis-**TYE**-tis): An inflammation of the lacrimal sac that is associated with faulty tear drainage.

deafness: The complete or partial loss of the ability to hear.

decubitus (dee-**KYOU**-bih-tus): The act of lying down or the position assumed in lying down.

dehydration: A condition in which fluid loss exceeds fluid intake and disrupts the body's normal electrolyte balance.

delirium (dah-**LEER**-ee-um): A potentially reversible condition often associated with a high fever that comes on suddenly in which the patient is confused, disoriented, and unable to think clearly.

delirium tremens (dah-**LEER**-ee-um **TREE**-mens): A form of acute organic brain syndrome due to alcohol withdrawal that is characterized by sweating, tremor, restlessness, anxiety, mental confusion, and hallucinations.

delusion (dee-**LOO**-zhun): A false personal belief that is maintained despite obvious proof or evidence to the contrary.

dementia (dee-**MEN**-shee-ah): A slowly progressive decline in mental abilities including impaired memory, thinking, and judgment.

dental calculus (**KAL**-kyou-luhs): Hardened dental plaque on the teeth that irritates the surrounding tissues.

dental caries (**KAYR**-eez): An infectious disease that destroys the enamel and dentin of the tooth; also known as tooth decay or a cavity.

dental plaque (**PLACK**): A soft deposit consisting of bacteria and bacterial by-products that builds up on the teeth and is a major cause of dental caries and periodontal disease.

dermatitis (**der**-mah-**TYE**-tis): Inflammation of the upper layers of skin.

dermatitis, contact: A localized allergic response caused by contact with an irritant or allergen that causes redness, itching, and rash.

dermatomycosis (der-mah-toh-my-**KOH**-sis): A fungal infection that causes white to light brown areas on the skin; also known as tinea versicolor.

dermatopathy (**der**-mah-**TOP**-ah-thee): Any disease of the skin.

dermatosis (der-mah-**TOH**-sis): A general term used to denote any skin lesion or group of lesions, or eruptions of any type that is *not* associated with inflammation.

detached retina: The retina is pulled away from its normal position of being attached to the choroid in the back of the eye.

developmental disorder: An anomaly or malformation that is present at birth.

diabetes insipidus (dye-ah-**BEE**-teez in-**SIP**-ih-dus): A condition caused by insufficient production of the antidiuretic hormone (ADH) or by the inability of the kidneys to respond to ADH that allows too much fluid to be excreted.

diabetes mellitus (dye-ah-**BEE**-teez mel-**EYE**-tus *or* **MEL**-ih-tus): A group of metabolic diseases characterized by hyperglycemia resulting from defects in insulin secretion, insulin action, or both.

diabetes mellitus, gestational: A form of diabetes that may occur during pregnancies and usually disappears after delivery.

diabetes mellitus, type 1: An insulin deficiency disorder; also known as insulin-dependent diabetes mellitus.

diabetes mellitus, type 2: An insulin resistance disorder; also known as non–insulin-dependent diabetes mellitus.

diabetic ketoacidosis (**kee**-toh-**ass**-ih-**DOH**-sis): An acute, life-threatening complication is caused by a severe insulin deficiency.

diabetic nephropathy: Disease of the kidney caused by long-term diabetes mellitus.

diaphoresis (dye-ah-foh-**REE**-sis): Profuse sweating.

diarrhea (**dye**-ah-**REE**-ah): Abnormal frequency of loose or watery stools.

diphtheria (dif-**THEE**-ree-ah): An acute infectious disease of the throat and upper respiratory tract caused by the presence of diphtheria bacteria.

diplopia (dih-**PLOH**-pee-ah): The perception of two images of a single object; also known as double vision.

diuresis (dye-you-**REE**-sis): Increased excretion of urine.

diverticulitis (dye-ver-tick-you-**LYE**-tis): Inflammation of one or more diverticulum.

Down syndrome: A genetic syndrome characterized by varying degrees of mental retardation and multiple physical abnormalities; also known as trisomy 21.

Duchenne's muscular dystrophy (doo-**SHENZ**): A severe form of muscular dystrophy that appears between 2 and 6 years of age.

ductal carcinoma in situ: Breast cancer at its earliest stage before the cancer has broken through the wall of the duct.

duodenal ulcers (dew-oh-**DEE**-nal *or* dew-**ODD**-eh-nal UL-serz): Peptic ulcers occurring in the upper part of the small intestine.

dyschromia (dis-**KROH**-mee-ah): Any disorder of the pigmentation of the skin or hair.

dyscrasia (dis-**KRAY**-zee-ah): Any abnormal or pathologic condition of the blood.

dyskinesia (**dis**-kih-**NEE**-zee-ah): Distortion or impairment of voluntary movement as in a tic or spasm.

dyslexia (dis-**LECK**-see-ah): A learning disability characterized by reading achievement that falls substantially below that expected given the individual's chronological age, measured intelligence, and age-appropriate education.

dysmenorrhea (**dis**-men-oh-**REE**-ah): Abdominal pain caused by uterine cramps during a menstrual period.

dyspepsia (dis-**PEP**-see-ah): An impairment of digestion; also known as indigestion.

dysphagia (dis-**FAY**-jee-ah): Difficulty in swallowing.

dysphonia (dis-**FOH**-nee-ah): Any voice impairment including hoarseness, weakness, or loss of voice.

dysplasia (dis-**PLAY**-see-ah): Abnormal development or growth of cells.

dysplasia, cervical: The abnormal growth of cells of the cervix; also known as precancerous lesions.

dyspnea (**DISP**-nee-ah): Difficult or labored breathing; also known as shortness of breath.

dysrhythmia (dis-**RITH**-mee-ah): An irregularity or the loss of normal rhythm of the heartbeat; also known as cardiac arrhythmia.

dystaxia (dis-**TACK**-see-ah): Difficulty in controlling voluntary movement; also known as partial ataxia.

dystonia (dis-**TOH**-nee-ah): Condition of abnormal muscle tone.

dysuria (dis-**YOU**-ree-ah): Difficult or painful urination.

E

E. coli: An intestinal infection caused by *Escherichia coli.*

ecchymosis (**eck**-ih-**MOH**-sis): A purplish area caused by bleeding within the skin; also known as a bruise.

eclampsia (eh-**KLAMP**-see-ah): A more serious form of preeclampsia characterized by convulsions and sometimes coma.

ectopic pregnancy (eck-**TOP**-ick): A pregnancy in which the fertilized egg is implanted and begins to develop outside of the uterus; also known as an extrauterine pregnancy.

ectropion (eck-**TROH**-pee-on): The turning outward of the edge of the eyelid.

eczema (**ECK**-zeh-mah): An acute or chronic skin inflammation characterized by erythema, papules, vesicles, pustules, scales, crusts, scabs, and possibly itching.

edema (eh-**DEE**-mah): Excess fluid in body tissues, causing swelling.

effusion (eh-**FEW**-zhun): The escape of fluid from blood or lymphatic vessels into the tissues or a cavity.

effusion, pleural: Abnormal escape of fluid into the pleural cavity that prevents the lung from fully expanding.

emaciated (ee-**MAY**-shee-ayt-ed): Abnormally thin.

embolism (**EM**-boh-lizm): Blockage of a vessel by an embolus.

embolus (**EM**-boh-lus): A foreign object, such as a blood clot, quantity of air or gas, or a bit of tissue or tumor that is circulating in the blood.

emesis (**EM**-eh-sis): To expel the contents of the stomach through the esophagus and out of the mouth; also known as vomiting.

emmetropia (em-eh-**TROH**-pee-ah): The normal relationship between the refractive power of the eye and the shape of the eye that enables light rays to focus correctly on the retina.

emphysema (**em**-fih-**SEE**-mah: The progressive loss of lung function due a decrease in the total number of alveoli, the enlargement of the remaining alveoli, and then the progressive destruction of their walls.

empyema (*em*-pye-**EE**-mah): An accumulation of pus in the pleural cavity; also known as pyothorax.

encephalitis (**en**-sef-ah-**LYE**-tis): Inflammation of the brain.

encephalocele (en-**SEF**-ah-loh-**seel**): A congenital gap in the skull with herniation of brain substance; also known as a craniocele.

encephalomalacia (en-**sef**-ah-loh-mah-**LAY**-shee-ah): Abnormal softening of the brain.

encephalopathy (en-**sef**-ah-**LOP**-ah-thee): Any degenerative disease of the brain.

endemic (en-**DEM**-ick): Ongoing presence of a disease within a population, group, or area.

endocarditis (**en**-doh-kar-**DYE**-tis): Inflammation of the inner layer of the heart.

endocarditis, bacterial: Inflammation of the inner lining or valves of the heart caused by bacteria.

endocervicitis (**en**-doh-**ser**-vih-**SIGH**-tis): Inflammation of the mucous membrane lining of the cervix.

endocrinopathy (**en**-doh-krih-**NOP**-ah-thee): Any disease due to a disorder of the endocrine system.

endometriosis (**en**-doh-**mee**-tree-**OH**-sis): A condition in which endometrial tissue escapes the uterus and grows on other structures in the pelvic cavity.

endometritis (**en**-doh-mee-**TRY**-tis): Inflammation of the endometrium.

enteritis (**en**-ter-**EYE**-tis): Inflammation of the small intestines.

entropion (en-**TROH**-pee-on): The turning inward of the edge of the eyelid.

enuresis (en-you-**REE**-sis): The involuntary discharge of urine.

epicondylitis (**ep**-ih-**kon**-dih-**LYE**-tis): Inflammation of the tissues surrounding the elbow.

epidemic (ep-ih-**DEM**-ick): Sudden and widespread outbreak of a disease within a population group or area.

epididymitis (**ep**-ih-did-ih-**MY**-tis): Inflammation of the epididymis.

epiglottitis (**ep**-ih-glot-**TYE**-tis): Inflammation of the epiglottis.

epilepsy (**EP**-ih-**lep**-see) is a group of neurologic disorders characterized by recurrent episodes of seizures.

epilepsy, grand mal (**GRAN MAHL EP**-ih-**lep**-see): The more severe form of epilepsy that is characterized by generalized tonic-clonic seizures.

epilepsy, petit mal (peh-**TEE MAHL EP**-ih-**lep**-see): The milder form of epilepsy in which there is a sudden, temporary loss of consciousness, lasting only a few seconds; also known as absence epilepsy.

epispadias (**ep**-ih-**SPAY**-dee-as): In the male, a congenital abnormality in which the urethral opening is located on the upper surface of the penis. In the female with epispadias, the urethral opening is in the region of the clitoris.

epistaxis (**ep**-ih-**STACK**-sis): Bleeding from the nose; also known as a nosebleed.

epithelioma (**ep**-ih-thee-lee-**OH**-mah): A benign or malignant tumor originating in the epidermis that may occur on the skin or mucous membranes.

eructation (eh-ruk-**TAY**-shun): The act of belching or raising gas orally from the stomach.

erythema (**er**-ih-**THEE**-mah): Any redness of the skin such as a nervous blush, an inflammation, or a mild sunburn.

erythrocytosis (eh-**rith**-roh-sigh-**TOH**-sis): An abnormal increase in the number of circulating red blood cells.

esophagalgia (eh-**sof**-ah-**GAL**-jee-ah): Pain in the esophagus.

esophageal reflux (eh-**sof**-ah-**JEE**-al **REE**-flucks): The upward flow of stomach acid into the esophagus; also known as gastroesophageal reflux disease.

esophageal varices (eh-**sof**-ah-**JEE**-al **VAYR**-ih-seez): Enlarged and swollen veins at the lower end of the esophagus.

esotropia (**es**-oh-**TROH**-pee-ah): Strabismus characterized by an inward deviation of one eye in relation to the other; also known as cross-eyes.

etiology (**ee**-tee-**OL**-oh-jee): Study of the causes of diseases.

eupnea (youp-**NEE**-ah): Easy or normal breathing.

eustachitis (**you**-stay-**KYE**-tis): Inflammation of the eustachian tube.

Ewing's sarcoma (**YOU**-ingz sar-**KOH**-mah): Cancer usually occurring in the diaphyses of long bones in the arms and legs of children or adolescents.

exophthalmos (**eck**-sof-**THAL**-mos): Abnormal protrusion of the eyes.

exostosis (**eck**-sos-**TOH**-sis): Benign growth on the surface of a bone.

exotropia (**eck**-soh-**TROH**-pee-ah): Strabismus characterized by the outward deviation of one eye relative to the other; also known as wall-eye.

exudate (**ECKS**-you-dayt): Accumulated fluid in a cavity that has penetrated through vessel walls into the adjoining tissue.

F

fasciitis (**fas**-ee-**EYE**-tis): Inflammation of a fascia.

fibrillation (**fih**-brih-**LAY**-shun): Rapid, random, and ineffetive contractions of the heart.

fibrillation, atrial: Condition in which the atria beat faster than the ventricles.

fibrillation, ventricular: The result of irregular contractions of the ventricles that is fatal unless reversed by electric defibrillation.

fibrocystic breast disease (figh-broh-**SIS**-tick): The presence of single or multiple cysts in the breasts.

fibroid: A benign tumor composed of muscle and fibrous tissue that occurs in the wall of the uterus; also known as a leiomyoma.

fibromyalgia syndrome (figh-broh-my-**AL**-jee-ah): A chronic disorder of unknown cause characterized by widespread aching pain, tender points, and fatigue.

fibrosis (figh-**BROH**-sis): The abnormal formation of fibrous tissue.

fissure: A groove or cracklike sore of the skin; normal folds in the contours of the brain.

flutter: A cardiac arrhythmia in which the atrial contractions are rapid but regular.

functional: A disorder in which there are no detectable physical changes to explain the symptoms being experienced by the patient.

furuncles (FYOU-rung-kuls): Large tender, swollen, areas caused by staphylococcal infection around hair follicles; also known as boils.

G

galactocele (gah-**LACK**-toh-seel): A cystic enlargement of the mammary gland containing milk; also known as a galactoma.

galactoma (gal-ack-**TOH**-mah): See galactocele.

gallstone: A hard deposit that forms in the gallbladder and bile ducts; also known as biliary calculus.

gangrene (GANG-green): Tissue death usually associated with a loss of circulation.

gastrodynia (gas-troh-**DIN**-ee-ah): Pain in the stomach.

gastroenteritis (gas-troh-en-ter-**EYE**-tis): Inflammation of the stomach and small intestine.

gastroenterocolitis (gas-troh-**en**-ter-oh-koh-**LYE**-tis): Inflammation of the stomach, small intestine, and large intestine.

gastroesophageal reflux disease: The upward flow of stomach acid into the esophagus; also known as esophageal reflux.

gastrorrhagia (gas-troh-**RAY**-jee-ah): Bleeding from the stomach.

gastrorrhea (gas-troh-**REE**-ah): Excessive flow of gastric secretions.

gastrorrhexis (gas-troh-**RECK**-sis): Rupture of the stomach.

gastrosis (gas-**TROH**-sis): Any abnormal condition of the stomach.

genital herpes (HER-peez): A highly contagious sexually transmitted disease caused by the herpes simplex virus.

genital warts: A highly contagious sexually transmitted disease caused by the *human papillomavirus.*

gigantism (jigh-**GAN**-tiz-em *or* **JIGH**-en-tiz-em): Abnormal overgrowth of the body caused by excessive secretion of the growth hormone *before* puberty.

gingivitis (jin-jih-**VYE**-tis): Inflammation of the gums that is the earliest stage of periodontal disease.

glaucoma (glaw-**KOH**-mah): Increased intraocular pressure that damages the optic nerve and may cause the loss of peripheral vision and eventually blindness.

glomerulonephritis (gloh-**mer**-you-loh-neh-**FRY**-tis): Inflammation of the kidney involving primarily the glomeruli.

glycosuria (**glye**-koh-**SOO**-ree-ah): The presence of glucose in the urine that is commonly caused by diabetes.

goiter (**GOI**-ter): An abnormal enlargement of the thyroid gland that produces a swelling in the front part of the neck; also known as thyromegaly.

gonorrhea (gon-oh-**REE**-ah): A highly contagious sexually transmitted disease caused by the bacteria *Neisseria gonorrhoeae*.

granulation tissue: Tissue that forms during the healing of a wound to create what will become scar tissue.

granuloma (gran-you-**LOH**-mah): A general term used to describe small knot-like swellings of granulation tissue.

Graves' disease (**GRAYVZ** dih-**ZEEZ**): An autoimmune disorder characterized by hyperthyroidism, goiter, and exophthalmos.

Guillain-Barré syndrome (gee-**YAHN**-bah-**RAY**): A condition characterized by rapidly worsening muscle weakness that may lead to temporary paralysis.

gynecomastia (**guy**-neh-koh-**MAS**-tee-ah): The condition of excessive mammary development in the male.

H

halitosis (hal-ih-**TOH**-sis): An unpleasant breath odor that may be caused by dental diseases, respiratory, or gastric disorders; also known as bad breath.

hallucination (hah-**loo**-sih-**NAY**-shun): A sense perception that has no basis in external stimulation.

hallux valgus (**HAL**-ucks **VAL**-guss): Abnormal enlargement of the joint at the base of the great toe; also known as a bunion.

hamstring injury: Strain or tear of the posterior femoral muscles.

Hashimoto's thyroiditis (hah-shee-**MOH**-tohz **thigh**-roi-**DYE**-tis): An autoimmune disorder in which the immune system mistakenly attacks thyroid tissue, setting up an inflammatory process that may progressively destroy the gland.

hearing loss, conductive: A hearing loss in which the outer or middle ear does not conduct sound vibrations to the inner ear normally.

hearing loss, noise-induced: Damage to sensitive hairlike cells of the inner ear caused by repeated exposure to very intense noise such as aircraft engines, noisy equipment, and loud music.

hearing loss, sensorineural: A hearing loss caused by problems affecting the inner ear; also known as nerve deafness.

hemangioma (hee-**man**-jee-**OH**-mah): A benign tumor made up of newly formed blood vessels.

hemangioma, strawberry: This dark reddish purple growth is a benign tumor made up of newly formed blood vessels that is usually present at birth; also known as a birthmark.

hematemesis (hee-mah-**TEM**-eh-sis *or* **hem**-ah-**TEM**-eh-sis): Vomiting blood.

hematoma (hee-mah-**TOH**-mah): A collection of blood trapped within tissues.

hematoma, cranial: A collection of blood trapped in the tissues of the brain.

hematoma, subungual: A collection of blood trapped in the tissues under a nail.

hematuria (hee-mah-**TOO**-ree-ah *or* **hem**-ah-**TOO**-ree-ah): The presence of blood in the urine.

hematuria, gross: Thepresence of blood in urine that can be detected without magnification.

hematuria, microscopic: The presence of blood in urine that can be seen only under a microscope.

hemianopia (hem-ee-ah-**NOH**-pee-ah): Blindness in one half of the visual field.

hemiparpesis (hem-ee-pah-**REE**-sis): Slight paralysis of one side of the body.

hemiplegia (hem-ee-**PLEE**-jee-ah): Paralysis of one side of the body.

hemochromatosis (hee-moh-**kroh**-mah-**TOH**-sis): A genetic disorder in which the intestines absorb too much iron and the excess accumulates in organs; also known as iron-overload disease.

hemophilia (hee-moh-**FILL**-ee-ah): A group of hereditary bleeding disorders in which one of the factors needed to clot the blood is missing.

hemoptysis (hee-**MOP**-tih-sis): Spitting of blood or blood-stained sputum derived from the lungs or bronchial tubes as the result of a pulmonary or bronchial hemorrhage.

hemorrhage (HEM-or-idj): The loss of a large amount of blood in a short time.

hemorrhoids (HEM-oh-roids): Enlarged veins in or near the anus that may cause pain and bleeding; also known as piles.

hemothorax (hee-moh-**THOH**-racks): An accumulation of blood in the pleural cavity.

hepatitis (hep-ah-**TYE**-tis): Inflammation of the liver.

hepatoenteric (hep-ah-toh-en-**TER**-ick): Referring to the liver and intestines.

hepatomegaly (hep-ah-toh-**MEG**-ah-lee): Abnormal enlargement of the liver.

hepatorrhexis (hep-ah-toh-**RECK**-sis): Rupture of the liver.

hereditary disorders: Diseases or conditions caused by a defective gene.

hernia (HER-nee-ah): Protrusion of a part or structure through the tissues normally containing it.

hernia, hiatal: Protrusion of part of the stomach through the esophageal sphincter in the diaphragm.

hernia, inguinal: Protrusion of a small loop of bowel through a weak place in the lower abdominal wall or groin.

herniated disk (HER-nee-**ayt**-ed): Rupture of the intervertebral disk resulting in pressure on spinal nerve roots; also known as a ruptured disk.

herpes labialis (HER-peez **lay**-bee-**AL**-iss): Blister-like sores caused by the herpes simplex virus that occur on the lips and adjacent tissue; also known as cold sores or fever blisters.

herpes zoster (**HER**-peez **ZOS**-ter): An acute viral infection characterized by painful skin eruptions that follow the underlying route of the inflamed nerve; also known as shingles.

hirsutism (**HER**-soot-izm): Abnormal hairiness; the appearance of male body or facial hair patterns in the female.

Hodgkin's lymphoma (**HODJ**-kinz): A form of lymphoma distinguished by the presence of Reed-Sternberg cells.

hordeolum (hor-**DEE**-oh-lum): An infection of one or more glands at the border of the eyelid; also known as a stye.

human immunodeficiency virus: A bloodborne pathogen that invades and then progressively impairs or kills cells of the immune system; also known as HIV.

human papilloma virus (**pap**-ih-**LOH**-mah): A highly contagious sexually transmitted disease caused by the human papillomavirus; also known as genital warts.

Huntington's disease: A hereditary disorder with symptoms that first appear in midlife and cause the irreversible and progressive loss of muscle control and mental ability; also known as Huntington's chorea.

hydrocele (**HIGH**-droh-seel): A hernia filled with fluid in the testicles or the tubes leading from the testicles.

hydrocephalus (high-droh-**SEF**-ah-lus): An abnormally increased amount of cerebrospinal fluid within the brain.

hydronephrosis (**high**-droh-neh-**FROH**-sis): Dilation of the renal pelvis of one or both kidneys.

hydroureter (**high**-droh-you-**REE**-ter): Distention of the ureter with urine that cannot flow because the ureter is blocked.

hyperalbuminemia (**high**-per-al-**byou**-mih-**NEE**-mee-ah): Abnormally high level of albumin in the blood.

hypercalcemia (**high**-per-kal-**SEE**-mee-ah): A condition characterized by abnormally high concentrations of calcium circulating in the blood instead of being stored in the bones.

hypercrinism (**high**-per-**KRY**-nism): A condition caused by excessive secretion of any gland, especially an endocrine gland.

hyperemesis (**high**-per-**EM**-eh-sis): Excessive vomiting.

hyperesthesia (**high**-per-es-**THEE**-zee-ah): A condition of excessive sensitivity to stimuli.

hyperglycemia (**high**-per-glye-**SEE**-mee-ah): An abnormally high concentration of glucose in the blood.

hyperglycosuria (**high**-per-**glye**-koh-**SOO**-ree-ah): Presence of excess sugar in the urine.

hypergonadism (**high**-per-**GOH**-nad-izm): The condition of excessive secretion of hormones by the sex glands.

hyperhidrosis (**high**-per-high-**DROH**-sis): The condition of excessive sweating.

hyperinsulinism (**high**-per-**IN**-suh-lin-izm): A condition marked by excessive secretion of insulin that produces hypoglycemia.

hyperkinesia (high-per-kih-**NEE**-zee-ah): Abnormally increased motor function or activity; also known as hyperactivity.

hyperlipemia (high-per-lih-**PEE**-mee-ah). A general term for elevated plasma concentrations of cholesterol, triglycerides, and lipoproteins; also known as hyperlipidemia.

hyperlipidemia (high-per-**lip**-ih-**DEE**-mee-ah): See hyperlipemia.

hyperopia (high-per-**OH**-pee-ah): A defect in which light rays focus beyond the retina; also known as farsightedness.

hyperparathyroidism (high-per-**par**-ah-**THIGH**-roid-izm): Overproduction of parathyroid hormone that causes hypercalcemia and may lead to weakened bones and the formation of kidney stones.

hyperpituitarism (high-per-pih-**TOO**-ih-tah-rizm): Pathology that results in the excessive secretion by the anterior lobe of the pituitary gland.

hyperplasia (high-per-**PLAY**-zee-ah): An abnormal increase in the number of normal cells in normal arrangement in a tissue.

hyperpnea (high-perp-**NEE**-ah): An abnormal increase in the depth and rate of the respiratory movements.

hyperproteinuria (high-per-**proh**-tee-in-**YOU**-ree-ah): Presence of excess of protein in the urine.

hypertension: Consistent abnormally elevated blood pressure levels.

hyperthyroidism (high-per-**THIGH**-roid-izm): A condition of excessive thyroid hormones in the blood.

hypertonia (high-per-**TOH**-nee-ah): Condition of excessive tone of the skeletal muscles with increased resistance of muscle to passive stretching.

hyperventilation (high-per-ven-tih-**LAY**-shun): Abnormally rapid deep breathing, resulting in decreased levels of carbon dioxide at the cellular level.

hypocalcemia (high-poh-kal-**SEE**-mee-ah): A condition characterized by abnormally low levels of calcium in the blood.

hypochondriasis (high-poh-kon-**DRY**-ah-sis): A preoccupation with fears of having, or the idea that one has, a serious disease based on misinterpretation of one or more bodily signs or symptoms.

hypocrinism (high-poh-**KRY**-nism): A condition caused by deficient secretion of any gland, especially an endocrine gland.

hypoglycemia (high-poh-glye-**SEE**-mee-ah): An abnormally low concentration of glucose in the blood.

hypogonadism (high-poh-**GOH**-nad-izm): The condition of deficient secretion of hormones by the sex glands.

hypohidrosis (high-poh-high-**DROH**-sis): Abnormal condition resulting in the diminished flow of perspiration.

hypokinesia (high-poh-kIH-**NEE**-zee-ah): Abnormally decreased motor function or activity.

hypomenorrhea (high-poh-men-oh-**REE**-ah): A small amount of menstrual flow during a shortened regular menstrual period.

hypoparathyroidism (**high**-poh-**par**-ah-**THIGH**-roid-izm): A condition caused by an insufficient or absent secretion of the parathyroid glands.

hypoperfusion (**high**-poh-per-**FYOU**-zhun): A deficiency of blood passing through an organ or body part.

hypopituitarism (**high**-poh-pih-**TOO**-ih-tah-**rizm**): A condition of reduced secretion due to the partial or complete loss of the function of the anterior lobe of the pituitary gland.

hypoplasia (**high**-poh-**PLAY**-zee-ah): Incomplete development of an organ or tissue, but less severe in degree than aplasia.

hypopnea (**high**-poh-**NEE**-ah): Shallow or slow respiration.

hypospadias (**high**-poh-**SPAY**-dee-as): In the male, a congenital abnormality in which the urethral opening is on the undersurface of the penis. In the female with hypospadias the urethral opening is into the vagina.

hypotension (**high**-poh-**TEN**-shun): Lower than normal blood pressure.

hypothyroidism (**high**-poh-**THIGH**-roid-izm): A deficiency of thyroid secretion; also known as an underactive thyroid.

hypotonia (**high**-poh-**TOH**-nee-ah): Condition of diminished tone of the skeletal muscles with decreased resistance of muscle to passive stretching.

hypoxia (high-**POCK**-see-ah): Subnormal oxygen levels in the cells that is less severe than anoxia.

hysterocele (**HISS**-ter-oh-seel): Hernia of the uterus, particularly during pregnancy.

hysterorrhexis (**hiss**-ter-oh-**RECK**-sis): Rupture of the uterus, particularly during pregnancy.

I

iatrogenic (eye-**at**-roh-**JEN**-ick): An unfavorable response to medical treatment for a different disorder.

icterus (**ICK**-ter-us): Yellow discoloration of the skin and other tissues caused by greater than normal amounts of bilirubin in the blood; also known as jaundice.

ileitis (**ill**-ee-**EYE**-tis): Inflammation of the ileum.

ileus (**ILL**-ee-us): A temporary stoppage of intestinal peristalsis.

immunodeficiency (**im**-you-noh-deh-**FISH**-en-see): A condition that occurs when one or more parts of the immune system are deficient or missing.

impacted cerumen: An accumulation of ear wax that forms a solid mass adhering to the walls of the external auditory canal.

impetigo (**im**-peh-**TYE**-goh): A highly contagious bacterial skin infection characterized by isolated pustules that become crusted and rupture.

impingement syndrome (im-**PINJ**-ment): Inflammation of tendons that get caught in the narrow space between the bones within the shoulder joint.

impotence (**IM**-poh-tens): The inability of the male to achieve or maintain a penile erection; also known as erectile dysfunction.

incontinence (in-**KON**-tih-nents): The inability to control excretory functions.

incontinence, bowel: The inability to control the excretion of feces.

incontinence, urinary: The inability to control the voiding of urine.

infarct (IN-farkt): Localized area of necrosis (tissue death) caused by an interruption of the blood supply.

infectious mononucleosis (mon-oh-new-klee-**OH**-sis): An infection caused by the Epstein-Barr virus (one of the herpes viruses) that is characterized by fever, a sore throat, and enlarged lymph nodes.

infertility: The inability of a couple to achieve pregnancy after 1 year of regular, unprotected intercourse or the inability of a woman to carry a pregnancy to a live birth.

infestation: The dwelling of a parasite on external surface tissue.

inflammation (in-flah-**MAY**-shun): A localized response to injury or destruction of tissues.

influenza (in-flew-**EN**-zah): An acute, highly contagious viral respiratory infection, that is spread by respiratory droplets and occurs most commonly during the colder months.

insomnia: The prolonged or abnormal inability to sleep.

insulinemia (in-suh-lih-**NEE**-mee-ah): Abnormally high levels of insulin in the blood.

insulinoma (in-suh-lin-**OH**-mah): A benign tumor of the pancreas that causes hypoglycemia.

intermittent claudication (klaw-dih-**KAY**-shun): A complex of symptoms including cramplike pain of the leg muscles caused by poor circulation.

interstitial cystitis (in-ter-**STISH**-al sis-**TYE**-tis): Inflammation within the wall of the bladder.

intestinal adhesions (ad-**HEE**-zhunz): Abnormally held together parts of the intestine where they normally should be separate.

intestinal obstruction: A complete stoppage or serious impairment to the passage of the intestinal contents.

intussusception (in-tus-sus-**SEP**-shun): Telescoping of one part of the intestine into the opening of an immediately adjacent part.

invasive ductal carcinoma: A form of breast cancer that starts in the milk duct, breaks through the wall of that duct, and invades fatty breast tissue; also known as infiltrating ductal carcinoma.

invasive lobular carcinoma: Breast cancer that starts in the milk glands, breaks through the wall of the gland and invades the fatty tissue of the breast; also known as infiltrating lobular carcinoma.

iridalgia (ir-ih-**DAL**-jee-ah): Pain felt in the iris.

iridopathy (ir-ih-**DOP**-ah-thee): Any disease of the iris.

iritis (eye-**RYE**-tis): Inflammation of the iris.

irritable bowel syndrome: A disorder of the motility of the entire gastrointestinal tract characterized by abdominal pain, nausea, gas, constipation, and/or diarrhea; also known as spastic colon.

ischemia (iss-**KEE**-mee-ah): Deficiency in blood supply due to either the constriction or the obstruction of a blood vessel.

ischemic heart disease (iss-**KEE**-mick): A group of cardiac disabilities resulting from an insufficient supply of oxygenated blood to the heart.

J

jaundice (**JAWN**-dis): Yellow discoloration of the skin and other tissues caused by greater than normal amounts of bilirubin in the blood; also known as icterus.

K

Kaposi's sarcoma (**KAP**-oh-seez sar-**KOH**-mah): A form of sarcoma that is frequently associated with HIV and may affect the skin, mucous membranes, lymph nodes and internal organs.

keloid (**KEE**-loid): An abnormally raised or thickened scar that is usually smooth and shiny.

keratitis (**ker**-ah-**TYE**-tis): Inflammation of the cornea of the eye.

keratosis (**kerr**-ah-**TOH**-sis): Any skin condition in which there is overgrowth and thickening of the skin.

ketonuria (**kee**-toh-**NEW**-ree-ah): The presence of ketones in the urine.

kleptomania (**klep**-toh-**MAY**-nee-ah): A personality disorder characterized by a recurrent failure to resist impulses to steal objects not for immediate use or their monetary value.

koilonychia (**koy**-loh-**NICK**-ee-ah): A malformation of the nails that is often indicative of iron-deficiency anemia in which the outer surface is scooped out; also known as spoon nail.

kyphosis (kye-**FOH**-sis): Abnormal increase in the outward curvature of the thoracic spine as viewed from the side; also known as humpback or dowager's hump.

L

labyrinthitis (**lab**-ih-rin-**THIGH**-tis): Inflammation of the labyrinth resulting in vertigo.

laryngoplegia (**lar**-ing-goh-**PLEE**-jee-ah): Paralysis of the larynx.

laryngorrhagia (**lar**-ing-goh-**RAY**-jee-ah): Bleeding from the larynx.

laryngospasm (lah-**RING**-goh-spazm): A sudden spasmodic closure of the larynx.

leiomyoma (**lye**-oh-my-**OH**-mah): A benign tumor composed of muscle and fibrous tissue that occurs in the wall of the uterus; also known as a fibroid.

lesion (**LEE**-zhun): A pathologic change of the tissues due to disease or injury.

lethargy (**LETH**-ar-jee): A lowered level of consciousness marked by listlessness, drowsiness, and apathy.

leukemia (loo-**KEE**-mee-ah): A malignancy characterized by a progressive increase of abnormal leukocytes.

leukopenia (loo-koh-**PEE**-nee-ah): An abnormal decrease in the number of white blood cells.

leukorrhea (loo-koh-REE-ah): A profuse white mucus discharge from the uterus and vagina.

lipedema (lip-eh-**DEE**-mah): An abnormal swelling due to the collection of fat and fluid under the skin, usually between the calf and ankle.

lipoma (lih-**POH**-mah): A benign fatty deposit under the skin, causing a bump.

lochia (**LOH**-kee-ah): The vaginal discharge during the first week or two after childbirth.

lordosis (lor-**DOH**-sis): Abnormal increase in the forward curvature of the lower or lumbar spine; also known as swayback.

Lou Gehrig's disease: A degenerative disease of the motor neurons in which patients become progressively weaker until they are completely paralyzed; also known as amyotrophic lateral sclerosis.

lumbago (lum-**BAY**-goh): Pain of the lumbar region; also known as low back pain.

lupus erythematosus (**LOO**-pus er-ih-**thee**-mah-**TOH**-sus): An autoimmune disorder characterized by a red, scaly rash on the face and upper trunk.

luxation (luck-**SAY**-shun): Dislocation or displacement of a bone from its joint

lymphadenitis (lim-**fad**-eh-**NIGH**-tis): Inflammation of the lymph nodes; also known as swollen glands.

lymphadenopathy (lim-**fad**-eh-**NOP**-ah-thee): Any disease process usually involving enlargement of the lymph nodes.

lymphadenopathy, persistent generalized: The continued presence of enlarged lymph nodes that is often an indication of the presence of a malignancy or deficiency in immune system function.

lymphangioma (lim-**fan**-jee-**OH**-mah): A benign abnormal collection of lymphatic vessels forming a mass.

lymphangitis (lim-fan-**JIGH**-tis): Inflammation of the lymph vessel.

lymphedema (lim-feh-**DEE**-mah): An abnormal accumulation of fluid primarily in the legs and ankles that occurs when veins or lymph vessels do not drain properly.

lymphoma (lim-**FOH**-mah): A general term applied to malignancies that develop in the lymphatic system.

M

macular degeneration (**MACK**-you-lar): A gradually progressive condition that results in the loss of central vision but not in total blindness.

macule (**MACK**-youl): A discolored, flat spot such as a freckle or *flat* mole that is *less than* 1 cm in diameter.

major depressive episode: A prolonged period during which there is either a depressed mood or the loss of interest or pleasure in nearly all activities.

malaria (mah-**LAY**-ree-ah): A disease caused by a parasite that lives within certain mosquitoes and is transferred to humans by the bite of the mosquito.

malignant: Harmful, tending to spread, becoming progressively worse, and life-threatening.

malingering (mah-**LING**-ger-ing): The intentional creation of false or grossly exaggerated physical or psychological symptoms, motivated by external incentives such as avoiding work.

malnutrition: Lack of proper food or nutrients in the body, either due to a shortage of food or the improper absorption or distribution of nutrients.

manic episode: A distinct period during which there is an abnormally, and persistently elevated, expansive, and irritable mood.

mastitis (mas-**TYE**-tis): Inflammation of the breast usually associated with lactation but which may occur for other reasons.

mastodynia (**mas**-toh-**DIN**-ee-ah): Pain in the breast.

mastoiditis (**mas**-toy-**DYE**-tis): Inflammation of any part of the mastoid process.

measles: An acute, highly contagious viral disease transmitted by respiratory droplets that is characterized by Koplik's spots and a spreading skin rash.

meconium (meh-**KOH**-nee-um): A greenish material that collects in the intestine of a fetus and forms the first stools of a newborn.

melanodermatitis (**mel**-ah-noh-**der**-mah-**TYE**-tis): Excess melanin present in an area of skin inflammation.

melanoma, malignant: Skin cancer derived from cells capable of forming melanin.

melanosis (**mel**-ah-**NOH**-sis): Any condition of unusual deposits of black pigment in different parts of the body.

melasma: A pigmentation disorder characterized by brownish colored spots on the face; also known as chloasma or the mask of pregnancy.

melena (meh-**LEE**-nah *or* **MEL**-eh-nah): The passage of black stools containing digested blood.

Menière's syndrome (**men**-ee-**AYRZ** *or* men-**YEHRS**): A chronic disease of the inner ear characterized by three main symptoms: attacks of dizziness, a fluctuating hearing loss, and tinnitus.

meningitis (**men**-in-**JIGH**-tis): An inflammation of the meninges of the brain or spinal cord.

meningocele (meh-**NING**-goh-**seel**): The protrusion of the membranes of the brain or spinal cord through a defect in the skull or spinal column.

meningoencephalitis (meh-**ning**-goh-en-**sef**-ah-**LYE**-tis): Inflammation of the meninges and brain.

meningoencephalomyelitis (meh-**ning**-goh-en-**sef**-ah-loh-**my**-eh-**LYE**-tis): Inflammation of the meninges, brain, and spinal cord.

meningomalacia (meh-**ning**-goh-mah-**LAY**-shee-ah): Abnormal softening of the meninges.

menometrorrhagia (**men**-oh-**met**-roh-**RAY**-jee-ah): Excessive uterine bleeding occurring both during the menses and at irregular intervals.

menorrhagia (**men**-oh-**RAY**-jee-ah): An excessive amount of menstrual flow over a longer duration than a normal period.

mental retardation: Significantly below average general intellectual functioning that is accompanied by significant limitation in adaptive functioning.

metastasis (meh-**TAS**-tah-sis): A new cancer site that results from the spreading process.

metastasize (meh-**TAS**-tah-sighz): The process by which cancer spreads from one place to another.

metrorrhea (**mee**-troh-**REE**-ah): An abnormal uterine discharge.

metrorrhexis (**mee**-troh-**RECK**-sis): Rupture of the uterus.

migraine headache (**MY**-grayn): A syndrome characterized by sudden, severe, sharp headache usually present only on one side.

miliaria (mill-ee-**AYR**-ee-ah): Trapped sweat that produces a skin rash and itching; also known as heat rash or prickly heat.

mitral stenosis (steh-**NOH**-sis): Abnormal narrowing of the opening of the mitral valve.

mitral valve prolapse: Abnormal protrusion of the mitral value that results in the incomplete closure of the valve.

mittelschmerz (**MIT**-uhl-schmehrts): Pain between menstrual periods.

monochromatism (**mon**-oh-**KROH**-mah-tizm): The lack of the ability to distinguish colors; also known as color blindness.

multiple sclerosis (skleh-**ROH**-sis): A progressive autoimmune disorder characterized by scattered patches of demyelination of nerve fibers of the brain and spinal cord.

mumps: An acute viral disease characterized by swelling of the parotid glands. (The parotid glands are salivary glands located on the face just in front of the ears.)

Munchausen syndrome (**MUHN**-chow-zen): A condition in which the "patient" repeatedly makes up clinically convincing simulations of disease for the purpose of gaining medical attention.

Munchausen syndrome by proxy: A form of child abuse in which the abusive parent will falsify an illness in a child by making up or creating symptoms and then seeking medical treatment.

muscular dystrophy (**DIS**-troh-fee): A group of inherited muscle disorders that cause muscle weakness without affecting the nervous system.

myalgia (my-**AL**-jee-ah): Muscle tenderness or pain.

myasthenia (**my**-as-**THEE**-nee-ah): Muscle weakness from any cause.

myasthenia gravis (**my**-as-**THEE**-nee-ah **GRAH**-vis): An autoimmune disease in which there is an abnormality in the neuromuscular function causing episodes of muscle weakness.

mycoplasma pneumonia (**my**-koh-**PLAZ**-mah new-**MOH**-nee-ah): A milder but longer lasting form of the pneumonia caused by the fungi *Mycoplasma pneumoniae*; also known as walking pneumonia.

mycosis (my-**KOH**-sis): Any disease caused by a fungus.

myelitis (**my**-eh-**LYE**-tis): Inflammation of the spinal cord; also inflammation of bone marrow.

myeloma (**my**-eh-**LOH**-mah): A malignant tumor composed of cells derived from hemopoietic tissues of the bone marrow.

myelopathy (my-eh-**LOP**-ah-thee): Any pathologic condition of the spinal cord.

myelosis (**my**-eh-**LOH**-sis): A tumor of the spinal cord; also an abnormal proliferation of bone marrow tissue.

myocardial infarction (**my**-oh-KAR-dee-al in-**FARK**-shun): Occlusion of a coronary artery resulting in an infarct of the affected myocardium; also known as a heart attack.

myocarditis (**my**-oh-kar-**DYE**-tis): Inflammation of the myocardium.

myocele (**MY**-oh-seel): Protrusion of a muscle through its ruptured sheath or fascia.

myoclonus (**my**-oh-**KLOH**-nus *or* my-**OCK**-loh-nus): Spasm or twitching of a muscle or group of muscles.

myofascial damage (**my**-oh-**FASH**-ee-ahl): Tenderness and swelling of the muscles and their surrounding tissues that is caused by overworking the muscles.

myolysis (my-**OL**-ih-sis): Degeneration of muscle tissue.

myoma (my-**OH**-mah): A benign neoplasm made up of muscle tissue.

myomalacia (**my**-oh-mah-**LAY**-shee-ah): Abnormal softening of muscle tissue.

myonecrosis (**my**-oh-neh-**KROH**-sis): Death of individual muscle fibers.

myoparesis (**my**-oh-**PAR**-eh-sis): Weakness or slight paralysis of a muscle.

myopathy (my-**OP**-ah-thee): Any pathologic change or disease of muscle tissue.

myopia (my-**OH**-pee-ah): A defect in which light rays focus in front of the retina; also known as nearsightedness.

myorrhexis (**my**-oh-**RECK**-sis): Rupture of a muscle.

myosarcoma (**my**-oh-sahr-**KOH**-mah): A malignant tumor derived from muscle tissue.

myosclerosis (**my**-oh-skleh-**ROH**-sis): Abnormal hardening of muscle tissue.

myositis (**my**-oh-**SIGH**-tis): Inflammation of skeletal muscle tissue.

myotonia (**my**-oh-**TOH**-nee-ah): Delayed relaxation of a muscle after a strong contraction.

myringitis (**mir**-in-**JIGH**-tis): Inflammation of the tympanic membrane.

myxedema (**mick**-seh-**DEE**-mah): A severe form of hypothyroidism in adults.

N

narcissistic personality disorder (**nahr**-sih-**SIS**-tick): A pattern of an exaggerated needed for admiration and complete lack of empathy.

narcolepsy (**NAR**-koh-**lep**-see): A syndrome characterized by recurrent uncontrollable seizures of drowsiness and sleep.

nausea (**NAW**-see-ah): The sensation that leads to the urge to vomit.

neoplasm (**NEE**-oh-plazm): A new and abnormal tissue formation that may be benign or malignant; also known as a tumor.

nephrectasis (neh-**FRECK**-tah-sis): Distention of a kidney.

nephritis (neh-**FRY**-tis): Inflammation of the kidney.

nephrolith (**NEF**-roh-lith): Presence of stones in the kidney; also known as renal calculus or a kidney stone.

nephrolithiasis (**nef**-roh-lih-**THIGH**-ah-sis): A disorder characterized by the presence of stones in the kidney.

nephromalacia (**nef**-roh-mah-**LAY**-shee-ah): Abnormal softening of the kidney.

nephropathy (neh-**FROP**-ah-thee): Disease of the kidney.

nephroptosis (**nef**-rop-**TOH**-sis): The downward displacement of the kidney; also known as a floating kidney.

nephropyosis (**nef**-roh-pye-**OH**-sis): Formation or discharge of pus from the kidney.

nephrosclerosis (**nef**-roh-skleh-**ROH**-sis): Abnormal hardening of the kidney.

nephrosis (neh-**FROH**-sis): Any abnormal condition of the kidney.

nephrotic syndrome (neh-**FROT**-ick): A group of kidney diseases characterized by edema, hyperproteinuria, hypoproteinemia, and hyperlipidemia.

neuralgia (new-**RAL**-jee-ah): Pain in a nerve or nerves.

neuritis (new-**RYE**-tis): Inflammation of a nerve or nerves.

neuroblastoma (**new**-roh-blas-**TOH**-mah): A sarcoma of nervous system origin.

neuroma (new-**ROH**-mah): A benign tumor made up nerve tissue.

neuromalacia (**new**-roh-mah-**LAY**-shee-ah): Abnormal softening of a nerve or nerves.

nevi (**NEE**-vye): Small dark skin growths that develop from melanocytes in the skin; also known as moles.

nevi, dysplastic: Atypical moles that may develop into skin cancer.

nocturia (nock-**TOO**-ree-ah): Excessive urination during the night.

nocturnal enuresis: The involuntary discharge of urine during sleep; also known as bed-wetting.

nocturnal myoclonus (nock-**TER**-nal **my**-oh-**KLOH**-nus *or* my-**OCK**-loh-nus): Jerking of the limbs that may occur normally as a person is falling asleep.

nodule (**NOD**-youl): A small, solid bump that may be felt within the skin or may be raised as if it had formed below the surface of the skin and pushed upward.

non-Hodgkin's lymphomas: The term used to describe all lymphomas other than Hodgkin's lymphoma.

nosocomial (**nos**-oh-**KOH**-mee-al): A hospital-acquired infection that was not present on admission but appears 72 hours or more after hospitalization.

nulligravida (**null**-ih-**GRAV**-ih-dah): A woman who has never been pregnant.

nullipara (nuh-**LIP**-ah-rah): A woman who has never borne a viable child.

nyctalopia (**nick**-tah-**LOH**-pee-ah): A condition in which the individual has difficulty seeing at night; also known as night blindness.

nystagmus (nis-**TAG**-mus): Involuntary, constant, rhythmic movement of the eyeball.

O

obesity (oh-**BEE**-sih-tee): An excessive accumulation of fat in the body.

obsessions: Persistent ideas, thoughts, or images that cause the individual anxiety or distress.

obsessive-compulsive disorder: A pattern of specific behaviors, such as repeated handwashing, that are caused by obsessions and compulsions.

occlusion (ah-**KLOO**-zhun): Blockage in a canal, vessel, or passageway in the body; coming together.

oligomenorrhea (**ol**-ih-goh-**men**-oh-**REE**-ah): Markedly reduced menstrual flow and abnormally infrequent menstruation.

oligospermia (**ol**-ih-goh-**SPER**-mee-ah): An abnormally low number of sperm in the ejaculate; also known as a low sperm count.

oliguria (**ol**-ih-**GOO**-ree-ah): Scanty urination.

onychia (oh-**NICK**-ee-ah): Inflammation of the matrix of the nail; also known as onychitis.

onychitis (**on**-ih-**KYE**-tis): See onychia.

onychocryptosis (**on**-ih-koh-krip-**TOH**-sis): Ingrown toenail.

onychoma (**on**-ih-**KOH**-mah): A tumor arising from the nail bed.

onychomalacia (**on**-ih-koh-mah-**LAY**-shee-ah): Abnormal softening of the nails.

onychomycosis (**on**-ih-koh-my-**KOH**-sis): Any fungus infection of the nail.

onychophagia (**on**-ih-koh-**FAY**-jee-ah): Nail biting or eating.

oophoritis (**oh**-ahf-oh-**RYE**-tis): Inflammation of an ovary.

orchitis (or-**KYE**-tis): Inflammation of one or both testicles; also known as testitis.

organic (or-**GAN**-ick): A disorder in which there are pathologic physical changes that explain the symptoms being experienced by the patient.

ostealgia (**oss**-tee-**AL**-jee-ah): Pain linked to an abnormal condition within a bone.

osteitis (**oss**-tee-**EYE**-tis): Inflammation of bone.

osteitis deformans (**oss**-tee-**EYE**-tis dee-**FOR**-manz): A disease of unknown cause characterized by extensive bone destruction followed by abnormal bone repair; also known as Paget's disease.

osteoarthritis (**oss**-tee-oh-ar-**THRIGH**-tis): Form of arthritis commonly associated with aging; also known as wear-and-tear arthritis.

osteoarthropathy (**oss**-tee-oh-ar-**THROP**-ah-thee): Any disease involving the bones and joints.

osteochondroma (**oss**-tee-oh-kon-**DROH**-mah): Benign bone tumors that occur as growths on the surface of a bone that protrude as hard lumps covered with a cap of cartilage.

osteomalacia (**oss**-tee-oh-mah-**LAY**-shee-ah): Abnormal softening of bones due to disease.

osteomyelitis (**oss**-tee-oh-**my**-eh-**LYE**-tis): Inflammation of the bone and bone marrow.

osteonecrosis (**oss**-tee-oh-neh-**KROH**-sis): Death of bone tissue caused by an insufficient blood supply, infection, malignancy, or trauma.

osteoporosis (**oss**-tee-oh-poh-**ROH**-sis): Loss of bone density and an increase in bone porosity frequently associated with aging.

osteosarcoma (**oss**-tee-oh-sar-**KOH**-mah): A malignant tumor usually involving the upper shaft of long bones, the pelvis, or knee.

osteosclerosis (**oss**-tee-oh-skleh-**ROH**-sis): Abnormal hardening of bone.

otalgia (oh-**TAL**-gee-ah): Pain in the ear.

otitis (oh-**TYE**-tis): Inflammation of the ear

otitis externa: Inflammation of the outer ear.

otitis media, acute (oh-**TYE**-tis **MEE**-dee-ah): Inflammation of the middle ear usually associated with an upper respiratory infection that is most commonly seen in young children.

otitis media, purulent (**PYOU**-roo-lent): A buildup of pus within the middle ear.

otitis media, serous: A fluid buildup in the middle ear that may follow acute otitis media or be caused by obstruction of the eustachian tube.

otomycosis (**oh**-toh-my-**KOH**-sis): A fungal infection of the external auditory canal.

otopyorrhea (**oh**-toh-**pye**-oh-**REE**-ah): The flow of pus from the ear.

otorrhagia (**oh**-toh-**RAY**-jee-ah): Bleeding from the ear.

otosclerosis (**oh**-toh-skleh-**ROH**-sis): Ankylosis of the bones of the middle ear resulting in a conductve hearing loss.

P

Paget's disease (**PAJ**-its): Disease of unknown cause characterized by extensive bone destruction followed by abnormal bone repair; also known as osteitis deformans.

palpitation (**pal**-pih-**TAY**-shun): A pounding or racing heart.

pancreatalgia (**pan**-kree-ah-**TAL**-jee-ah): Pain in the pancreas.

pancreatitis (**pan**-kree-ah-**TYE**-tis): Inflammation of the pancreas.

pandemic (pan-**DEM**-ick): A disease outbreak occurring over a large geographic area, possibly worldwide.

panic attack: A mental state that includes intense feelings of apprehension, fearfulness, terror, and impending doom plus physical symptoms that include shortness of breath and heart palpitations.

papilledema (**pap**-ill-eh-**DEE**-mah): Swelling and inflammation of the optic nerve at the point of entrance through the optic disk; also known as choked disk.

papilloma (**pap**-ih-**LOH**-mah): A benign epithelial tumor that projects from the surrounding surface.

papule (**PAP**-youl): A small, solid, raised skin lesion that is less than 0.5 cm in diameter; also known as a pimple.

paralysis (pah-**RAL**-ih-sis): Loss of sensation and voluntary muscle movements through disease or injury to its nerve supply.

paraplegia (**par**-ah-**PLEE**-jee-ah): Paralysis of both legs and the lower part of the body.

parasite (**PAR**-ah-sight): A plant or animal that lives on or within another living organism at the expense of that organism.

paraspadias (**par**-ah-**SPAY**-dee-as): A congenital male abnormality in which the urethral opening is on one side of the penis.

paresthesia (**par**-es-**THEE**-zee-ah): An abnormal sensation, such as burning, tingling, or numbness, for no apparent reason.

Parkinson's disease: A chronic slowly progressive, degenerative, central nervous system disorder characterized by fine muscle tremors, a masklike facial expression, and a shuffling gait.

paronychia (**par**-oh-**NICK**-ee-ah): An acute or chronic infection of the skin fold at the margin of a nail.

paroxysm (**PAR**-ock-sizm): A sudden convulsion, seizure, or spasm.

paroxysmal (**par**-ock-**SIZ**-mal): Sudden or spasmlike.

paroxysmal tachycardia: A fast heartbeat of sudden onset.

pathogen (**PATH**-oh-jen): A microorganism that causes a disease.

pattern baldness, female: A condition in which the hair thins in the front and on the sides, and sometimes on the crown.

pattern baldness, male: A condition in which the hairline recedes from the front to the back until only a horseshoe-shaped area of hair remains in the back and temples.

patulous eustachian tube (**PAT**-you-lus): Distention of the eustachian tube.

pediculosis (pee-**dick**-you-**LOH**-sis): An infestation with lice.

pediculosis capitis: An infestation with head lice.

pediculosis corporis: An infestation with body lice.

pediculosis pubis: An infestation with lice in the pubic hair and pubic region.

pelvic inflammatory disease: Any inflammation of the female reproductive organs not associated with surgery or pregnancy; also known as PID.

peptic ulcer: A lesion of the mucous membranes of the digestive system caused by the bacterium *Helicobacter pylori*.

pericarditis (**pehr**-ih-kar-**DYE**-tis): Inflammation of the pericardium.

periodontal disease: Inflammation of the tissues that surround and support the teeth; also known as periodontitis.

periodontitis (**pehr**-ee-oh-don-**TYE**-tis): Inflammation of the tissues that surround and support the teeth; also known as periodontal disease.

periostitis (**pehr**-ee-oss-**TYE**-tis): Inflammation of the periosteum.

peripheral neuritis (new-**RYE**-tis): A painful condition of the nerves of the hands and feet due to peripheral nerve damage; also known as peripheral neuropathy.

peripheral neuropathy (new-**ROP**-ah-thee): See peripheral neuritis.

personality disorder: An enduring pattern of inner experience and behavior that deviates markedly from the expectations of the individual's culture.

pertussis (per-**TUS**-is): A contagious bacterial infection of the upper respiratory tract that is characterized by a paroxysmal cough; also known as whooping cough.

petechiae (pee-**TEE**-kee-ee): Small pinpoint hemorrhages; smaller versions of bruises.

pharyngitis (**far**-in-**JIGH**-tis): Inflammation of the pharynx; also known as a sore throat.

pharyngolaryngitis (fah-**ring**-goh-**lar**-in-**JIGH**-tis): Inflammation of both the pharynx and the larynx.

pharyngorrhagia (**far**-ing-goh-**RAY**-jee-ah): Bleeding from the pharynx.

pharyngorrhea (**far**-ing-goh-**REE**-ah): An abnormal discharge from the pharynx.

phenylketonuria (**fen**-il-**kee**-toh-**NEW**-ree-ah): A genetic disorder in which an essential digestive enzyme is missing.

pheochromocytoma (fee-oh-**kroh**-moh-sigh-**TOH**-mah): A benign tumor of the adrenal medulla that causes the gland to produce excess epinephrine.

phimosis (figh-**MOH**-sis): A narrowing of the opening of the foreskin so it cannot be retracted to expose the glans penis.

phlebitis (fleh-**BYE**-tis): Inflammation of a vein or veins.

phleborrhexis (**fleb**-oh-**RECK**-sis): Rupture of a vein.

phlebostenosis (**fleb**-oh-steh-**NOH**-sis): Abnormal narrowing of the lumen of a vein.

phlegm (**FLEM**): Thick mucus secreted by the tissues lining the respiratory passages.

phobia (**FOH**-bee-ah): A persistent irrational fear of a specific thing or situation. This fear is strong enough to cause avoidance of that thing or situation.

pica (**PYE**-kah): An eating disorder in which there is persistent eating of non-nutritional substances such as clay.

pinealoma (**pin**-ee-ah-**LOH**-mah): Tumor of the pineal gland.

pinealopathy (**pin**-ee-ah-**LOP**-ah-thee): Any disorder of the pineal gland.

pituitarism (pih-**TOO**-ih-tar-izm): Any disorder of pituitary function.

placenta previa (plah-**SEN**-tah **PREE**-vee-ah): Abnormal implantation of the placenta in the lower portion of the uterus.

plaque (**PLACK**): A solid raised area of skin that is different from the area around it and greater than 0.5 cm in diameter.

pleuralgia (ploor-**AL**-jee-ah): Pain in the pleura or in the side.

pleurisy (**PLOOR**-ih-see): Inflammation of the visceral and parietal pleura in the thoracic cavity.

pneumoconiosis (**new**-moh-**koh**-nee-**OH**-sis): An abnormal condition caused by dust in the lungs that usually develops after years of environmental or occupational contact.

Pneumocystis carinii **pneumonia** (**new**-moh-**SIS**-tis kah-**RYE**-nee-eye new-**MOH**-nee-ah): A form of pneumonia caused by an infection with the parasite *Pneumocystis carinii.*

pneumonia (new-**MOH**-nee-ah): Inflammation of the lungs in which the air sacs fill with pus and other liquid.

pneumonitis (**new**-moh-**NIGH**-tis): Inflammation of the lungs.

pneumorrhagia (**new**-moh-**RAY**-jee-ah): Bleeding from the lungs.

pneumothorax (**new**-moh-**THOR**-racks): An accumulation of air or gas in the pleural space causing the lung to collapse.

poliomyelitis (**poh**-lee-oh-**my**-eh-**LYE**-tis): A viral infection of the gray matter of the spinal cord that may result in paralysis.

polyarteritis (**pol**-ee-ar-teh-**RYE**-tis): Inflammation involving several arteries.

polyarthritis (**pol**-ee-ar-**THRIGH**-tis): Inflammation of more than one joint.

polycystic ovary syndrome: Enlargement of the ovaries caused by the presence of many cysts.

polydipsia (**pol**-ee-**DIP**-see-ah): Excessive thirst.

polymenorrhea (**pol**-ee-**men**-oh-**REE**-ah): Abnormally frequent menstruation.

polymyalgia (**pol**-ee-my-**AL**-jee-ah): Pain in several muscle groups.

polymyositis (**pol**-ee-**my**-oh-**SIGH**-tis): A chronic, progressive disease affecting the skeletal muscles that is characterized by muscle weakness and atrophy.

polyneuritis (**pol**-ee-new-**RYE**-tis): Inflammation affecting many nerves.

polyp (**POL**-ip): A general term describing a mushroom-like growth from the surface of a mucous membrane.

polyuria (**pol**-ee-**YOU**-ree-ah): Excessive urination.

port-wine stain: A large reddish purple discoloration of the face or neck that is present at birth and will not resolve without treatment; also known as a birthmark.

postpolio syndrome: Recurrence later in life of some polio symptoms in individuals who have had poliomyelitis and have recovered from it.

posttraumatic stress disorder: The development of symptoms such as sleep disorders and anxiety after a psychologically traumatic event such as witnessing a shooting, surviving a natural disaster, or being held as a hostage.

preeclampsia (**pree**-ee-**KLAMP**-see-ah): A complication of pregnancy characterized by hypertension, edema, and proteinuria; also known as toxemia of pregnancy.

premenstrual syndrome: Symptoms occurring within the 2-week period before menstruation; also known as PMS.

presbycusis (**pres**-beh-**KOO**-sis): A progressive hearing loss occurring in old age.

presbyopia (**pres**-bee-**OH**-pee-ah): Changes in the eyes that occur with aging.

proctalgia (prock-**TAL**-jee-ah): Pain in and around the anus and rectum.

prolactinoma (proh-**lack**-tih-**NOH**-mah): A benign tumor of the pituitary gland that causes it to produce too much prolactin; also known as a prolactin-producing adenoma.

prolapse (proh-**LAPS**): Downward placement.

prolapse of uterus: Falling or sinking down of the uterus until it protrudes through the vaginal opening.

prostatitis (pros-tah-**TYE**-tis): Inflammation of the prostate gland.

prostatomegaly (pros-tah-toh-**MEG**-ah-lee): Abnormal enlargement of the prostate gland that may be benign or malignant.

prostatorrhea (pros-tah-toh-**REE**-ah): An abnormal flow of prostatic fluid discharged through the urethra.

prostrate (PROS-trayt): To collapse or to be overcome with exhaustion.

proteinuria (proh-tee-in-**YOU**-ree-ah): An abnormally high level of serum protein in the urine.

pruritus (proo-**RYE**-tus): Itching.

pruritus vulvae (proo-**RYE**-tus **VUL**-vee): A condition of severe itching of the external female genitalia.

pseudophakia (soo-doh-**FAY**-kee-ah): An eye in which the natural lens is replaced with an intraocular lens.

psoriasis (soh-**RYE**-uh-sis): A chronic autoimmune disorder of the skin characterized by red papules covered with silvery scales that occur predominantly on the elbows, knees, scalp, back, and butocks.

psychotic disorder (sigh-**KOT**-ick): The derangement of personality, loss of contact with reality, and deterioration of normal social functioning.

pulmonary edema (eh-**DEE**-mah): An accumulation of fluid in lung tissues.

pulmonary fibrosis: The formation of scar tissue that replaces the pulmonary alveolar walls.

puncture wound: A deep hole made by a sharp object such as a nail.

purpura (PUR-pew-rah): A condition characterized by hemorrhage into the skin that causes spontaneous bruising.

purulent (PYOU-roo-lent): Producing or containing pus.

pustule (PUS-tyoul): A small, circumscribed elevation of the skin containing pus.

putrefaction (pyou-treh-**FACK**-shun): Decay that produces foul-smelling odors.

pyelitis (pye-eh-**LYE**-tis): Inflammation of the renal pelvis.

pyelonephritis (pye-eh-loh-neh-**FRY**-tis): Inflammation of the renal pelvis and of the kidney.

pyemia (pye-**EE**-mee-ah): Presence of pus-forming organisms in the blood.

pyoderma (pye-oh-**DER**-mah): Any pus-forming skin disease.

pyometritis (pye-oh-meh-**TRY**-tis): A pus-containing inflammation of the uterus.

pyosalpinx (pye-oh-**SAL**-pinks): An accumulation of pus in the fallopian tube.

pyothorax (pye-oh-**THOH**-racks): An accumulation of pus in the pleural cavity; also known as empyema.

pyromania (pye-roh-**MAY**-nee-ah): A personality disorder characterized by a recurrent failure to resist impulses to set fires.

pyrosis (pye-**ROH**-sis): Regurgitation of stomach acid upward into the esophagus; also known as heartburn.

pyuria (pye-**YOU**-ree-ah): The presence of pus in the urine.

Q

quadriplegia (**kwad**-rih-**PLEE**-jee-ah): Paralysis of all four extremities.

R

rabies (**RAY**-beez): An acute viral infection that may be transmitted to humans by the blood, tissue, or saliva of an infected animal.

radiculitis (rah-**dick**-you-**LYE**-tis): Inflammation of the root of a spinal nerve; also known as a pinched nerve.

rale (**RAHL**): An abnormal rattle or crackle-like respiratory sound heard while breathing in.

Raynaud's phenomenon (ray-**NOHZ**): Intermittent attacks of pallor (paleness), cyanosis (blue color), and redness of the fingers and toes.

reflux (**REE**-flucks): A backward or return flow.

refractive disorder: A condition in which the lens and cornea do not bend light so that it focuses properly on the retina.

regurgitation (ree-**gur**-jih-**TAY**-shun): The return of swallowed food into the mouth.

renal colic (**REE**-nal **KOLL**-ick): Acute pain in the kidney area caused by blockage during the passage of a kidney stone.

renal failure: Inability of the kidney or kidneys to perform their functions; also known as kidney failure.

renal failure, acute: Sudden onset of renal failure that is characterized by uremia.

renal failure, chronic: A progressive disease that may be caused by a variety of conditions.

restenosis: The condition in which an artery that has been opened by angioplasty becomes blocked again.

retinal tear: The retina develops a hole as it is pulled away from its normal position.

retinitis (**ret**-ih-**NIGH**-tis): Inflammation of the retina.

retinoblastoma (**ret**-ih-noh-blas-**TOH**-mah): A malignant tumor of childhood arising from cells of the retina of the eye.

retinopathy (**ret**-ih-**NOP**-ah-thee): Any disease of the retina.

retinopathy, diabetic: A complication of diabetics causing damage to the retina of the eye.

retroflexion (**ret**-roh-**FLECK**-shun): Abnormal tipping with the body of the uterus bent forming an angle with the cervix.

retroversion (**ret**-roh-**VER**-zhun): Abnormal tipping of the entire uterus backward, with the cervix pointing forward.

rhinitis (rye-**NIGH**-tis): Inflammation of the nose.

rhinophyma (**rye**-noh-**FIGH**-muh): Hyperplasia of the nose; also known as bulbous nose.

rhinorrhea (**rye**-noh-**REE**-ah): An excessive flow of mucus from the nose; also known as a runny nose.

rhonchus (**RONG**-kus): An added sound with a musical pitch occurring during inspiration or expiration that results from a partially obstructed airway; also known as wheezing.

rickets (**RICK**-ets): Bone disorder caused by calcium and vitamin D deficiencies in early childhood.

rosacea (roh-**ZAY**-shee-ah): A chronic condition of unknown cause that produces redness, tiny pimples, and broken blood vessels.

rotator cuff tendinitis (ten-dih-**NIGH**-tis): Inflammation of the tendons of the rotator cuff.

rubella (roo-**BELL**-ah): A viral infection characterized by fever and a diffuse, fine, red rash; also known as German measles or 3-day measles.

S

salmonella (**sal**-moh-**NEL**-ah): An intestinal infection caused by nontyphoidal *Salmonella*.

salpingitis (**sal**-pin-**JIGH**-tis): Inflammation of a fallopian tube; inflammation of the eustachian tube.

sarcoma (sar-**KOH**-mah): A malignant tumor that arises from connective tissue.

scabies (**SKAY**-beez): A skin infection caused by an infestation with the itch mite.

scale: A flaking or dry patch made up of excess dead epidermal cells.

schizophrenia (**skit**-soh-**FREE**-nee-ah): A psychotic disorder that is characterized by delusions, hallucinations, disorganized speech that is often incoherent, and disruptive or catatonic behavior.

sciatica (sigh-**AT**-ih-kah) Inflammation of the sciatic nerve that results in pain along the course of the nerve through the thigh and leg.

scleritis (skleh-**RYE**-tis): Inflammation of the sclera of the eye.

scleroderma (**sklehr**-oh-**DER**-mah *or* **skleer**-oh-**DER**-mah): An autoimmune disorder that causes abnormal tissue thickening usually starting on the hands, feet, or face.

scoliosis (**skoh**-lee-**OH**-sis): Abnormal lateral curvature of the spine.

scotoma (skoh-**TOH**-mah): Abnormal area of absent or depressed vision surrounded by an area of normal vision.

sebaceous cyst (seh-**BAY**-shus): A cyst of a sebaceous gland, containing yellow, fatty material.

seborrhea (**seb**-oh-**REE**-ah): Any of several common skin conditions in which there is an overproduction of sebum.

seborrheic dermatitis (**seb**-oh-**REE**-ick **der**-mah-**TYE**-tis): An inflammation of the upper layers of the skin, caused by seborrhea.

seborrheic keratosis (**seb**-oh-**REE**-ick **kerr**-ah-**TOH**-sis): A benign flesh-colored, brown or black skin tumor.

seizure (SEE-zhur): A sudden, violent, involuntary contraction of a group of muscles caused by a disturbance in brain function; also known as a convulsion.

seizure, generalized tonic-clonic: A loss of consciousness and tonic convulsions followed by clonic convulsions; also known as a generalized seizure. See also convulsion, tonic and convulsion, clonic.

seizure, localized: A state that begins with specific motor, sensory, or psychomotor phenomena without loss of consciousness; also known as a partial seizure.

septicemia (sep-tih-**SEE**-mee-ah): The presence of pathogenic microorganisms or their toxins in the blood; also known as blood poisoning.

sexually transmitted diseases: Diseases transmitted through sexual intercourse or other genital contact; also known as venereal diseases.

shin splint: Pain caused by the muscle tearing away from the tibia.

sigmoiditis (sig-moi-**DYE**-tis): Inflammation of the sigmoid colon.

silicosis (sill-ih-**KOH**-sis): A form of pneumoconiosis caused by silica dust or glass in the lungs; also known as grinder's disease.

singultus (sing-**GUL**-tus): Myoclonus of the diaphragm that causes the characteristic hiccup sound with each spasm; also known as hiccups.

sinusitis (sigh-nuh-**SIGH**-tis): Inflammation of the sinuses.

skin tags: Small flesh-colored or light brown growths that hang from the body by fine stalks.

sleep apnea syndromes: A group of potentially deadly disorders in which breathing repeatedly stops during sleep for long enough periods to cause a measurable decrease in blood oxygen levels.

smoker's respiratory syndrome: A group of symptoms seen in smokers that include a cough, wheezing, vocal hoarseness, pharyngitis, difficult breathing, and susceptibility to respiratory infections.

somatoform (soh-**MAT**-oh-**form**): The presence of physical symptoms that suggest general medical conditions but are not explained by the patient's actual medical condition.

somnambulism (som-**NAM**-byou-lizm): The condition of walking without awakening; also known as sleepwalking.

somnolence (SOM-noh-lens): A condition of unnatural sleepiness or semiconsciousness approaching coma; however, a somnolent person can usually be aroused by verbal stimuli.

spasm: A sudden, violent, involuntary contraction of a muscle or a group of muscles; also known as a cramp.

spasmodic torticollis (spaz-**MOD**-ick **tor**-tih-**KOL**-is): A stiff neck due to spasmodic contraction of the neck muscles that pull the head toward the affected side; also known as wryneck.

spina bifida (SPY-nah **BIF**-ih-dah): A congenital defect in which the spinal canal fails to close around the spinal cord.

splenitis (splee-**NIGH**-tis): Inflammation of the spleen.

splenomegaly (splee-noh-**MEG**-ah-lee): Abnormal enlargement of the spleen.

splenorrhagia (**splee**-noh-**RAY**-jee-ah): Bleeding from the spleen.

spondylitis (**spon**-dih-**LYE**-tis): Inflammation of the vertebrae.

spondylolisthesis (**spon**-dih-loh-liss-**THEE**-sis): Forward movement of the body of one of the lower lumbar vertebra on the vertebra below it or on the sacrum.

spondylosis (**spon**-dih-**LOH**-sis): Any degenerative condition of the vertebrae.

sprain: Injury to a joint such as an ankle, knee, or wrist involving stretched or torn ligaments.

stillbirth: A fetus that died before or during delivery.

stoma (**STOH**-mah): An opening on a body surface that can occur naturally or may be created surgically.

strabismus (strah-**BIZ**-mus): A disorder in which the eyes cannot be directed in a parallel manner toward the same object.

strain: Injury to the body of the muscle or attachment of the tendon.

stricture: An abnormal band of tissue narrowing a body passage.

stridor (**STRYE**-dor): An abnormal, high-pitched, harsh or crowing sound heard during inspiration that results from a partial blockage of the pharynx, larynx, and trachea.

stroke: Damage to the brain that occurs when the blood flow to the brain is disrupted because a blood vessel supplying it is either blocked or has ruptured.

stroke, hemorrhagic (**hem**-oh-**RAJ**-ick): Damage to brain tissue caused by the rupture of leaking of a blood vessel within brain; also known as a bleed.

stroke, ischemic: Damage to the brain caused by narrowing or blockage of the carotid artery and the resulting decreased flow of blood to the brain; also known as a cerebrovascular accident.

stupor (**STOO**-per): A state of impaired consciousness marked by a lack of responsiveness to environmental stimuli.

subluxation (**sub**-luck-**SAY**-shun): Partial displacement of a bone from its joint.

sudden infant death syndrome: The unexplainable death of an apparently healthy infant that typically occurs while the infant is sleeping; also known as SIDS or crib death.

suppuration (**sup**-you-**RAY**-shun): Formation or discharge of pus.

syncope (**SIN**-koh-pee): The brief loss of consciousness caused by brief lack of oxygen in the brain; also known as fainting.

synechia (sigh-**NECK**-ee-ah): An adhesion that binds the iris to any adjacent structure.

synovitis (sin-oh-**VYE**-tiss): Inflammation of the synovial membrane that results in swelling and pain.

syphilis (**SIF**-ih-lis): A highly contagious sexually transmitted disease caused by the spirochete *Treponema pallidum*.

T

tachycardia (**tack**-ee-**KAR**-dee-ah): An abnormally fast heartbeat.

tachypnea (**tack**-ihp-**NEE**-ah): An abnormally rapid rate of respiration usually more than 20 breaths per minute.

talipes (**TAL**-ih-peez): Congenital deformity in which the foot may be turned outward or inward; also known as a clubfoot.

tardive dyskinesia (**TAHR**-div **dis**-kih-**NEE**-zee-ah): Late appearance of dyskinesia as a side effect of long-term treatment with certain antipsychotic drugs.

Tay-Sachs disease: A hereditary disease marked by progressive physical degeneration, mental retardation, and early death.

temporomandibular disorders (tem-poh-roh-man-**DIB**-you-lar): A group of complex symptoms related to the malfunctioning of the temporomandibular joint; also known as myofascial pain dysfunction.

tenalgia (ten-**AL**-jee-ah): Pain in a tendon; also known as tenodynia.

tendinitis (**ten**-dih-**NIGH**-tis): Inflammation of the tendons caused by excessive or unusual use of the joint; is also known as tendonitis.

tendonitis (**ten**-doh-**NIGH**-it is): See tendinitis.

tenodynia (**ten**-oh-**DIN**-ee-ah): Pain in a tendon; also known as tenalgia.

testitis (test-**TYE**-tis): Inflammation of one or both testicles; also known as orchitis.

tetanus (**TET**-ah-nus): An acute and potentially fatal bacterial infection of the central nervous system caused by the tetanus bacillus.

tetany (**TET**-ah-nee): An abnormal condition characterized by periodic painful muscle spasms and tremors.

thalassemia (thal-ah-**SEE**-mee-ah): A group of genetic disorders characterized by short-lived red blood cells that lack the normal ability to produce hemoglobin; also known as Cooley's anemia.

thrombocytopenia (**throm**-boh-**sigh**-toh-**PEE**-nee-ah): An abnormal decrease in the number of platelets; also known as thrombopenia.

thrombopenia: An abnormal decrease in the number of platelets; also known as thrombocytopenia.

thrombosis (throm-**BOH**-sis): An abnormal condition in which a thrombus develops within a blood vessel.

thrombotic occlusion (throm-**BOT**-ick ah-**KLOO**-zhun): Blocking of an artery by a clot.

thrombus (**THROM**-bus): A blood clot attached to the interior wall of a vein or artery.

thymitis (thigh-**MY**-tis): Inflammation of the thymus gland.

thymoma (thigh-**MOH**-mah): A benign tumor originating in the thymus.

thymopathy (thigh-**MOP**-ah-thee): Any disease of the thymus gland.

thyroiditis (thigh-roi-**DYE**-tis): Inflammation of the thyroid gland.

thyromegaly (**thigh**-roh-**MEG**-ah-lee): An abnormal enlargement of the thyroid gland that produces a swelling in the front part of the neck; also known as goiter.

thyrotoxicosis (**thy**-roh-**tock**-sih-**KOH**-sis): A life-threatening condition resulting from the presence of excessive quantities of the thyroid hormones; also known as thyroid storm.

tic douloureux (TICK doo-loo-**ROO**): Inflammation of the trigeminal nerve that is characterized by sudden, intense, sharp pain on one side of the face; also known as trigeminal neuralgia.

tinea (TIN-ee-ah): A fungus skin disease affecting different areas of the body; also known as ringworm.

tinea capitis: A fungal infection found on the scalps of children.

tinea cruris: A fungal infection of the genital area; also known as jock itch.

tinea pedis: A fungal infection found between the toes and on the feet; also known as athlete's foot.

tinnitus (tih-**NIGH**-tus): A ringing, buzzing, or roaring sound in the ears.

tonsillitis (ton-sih-**LYE**-tis): Inflammation of the tonsils.

toxemia of pregnancy: A complication of pregnancy characterized by hypertension, edema, and proteinuria; also known as preeclampsia.

tracheitis (tray-kee-**EYE**-tis): Inflammation of the trachea.

tracheorrhagia (tray-kee-oh-**RAY**-jee-ah): Bleeding from the trachea.

tracheostenosis (tray-kee-oh-steh-**NOH**-sis): Abnormal narrowing of the lumen of the trachea.

transient ischemic attack (iss-**KEE**-mick): The temporary interruption in the blood supply to the brain that may be a warning of an impending stroke.

trauma (TRAW-mah): Wound or injury.

trichomonas (trick-oh-**MOH**-nas): A vaginal inflammation caused by the protozoan parasite *Trichomonas vaginalis*.

tricuspid stenosis: Abnormal narrowing of the opening of the tricuspid valve.

trigeminal neuralgia: Inflammation of the trigeminal nerve that is characterized by sudden, intense, sharp pain on one side of the face; also known as tic douloureux.

tuberculosis (too-**ber**-kew-**LOH**-sis): An infectious disease caused by *Mycobacterium tuberculosis* that usually attacks the lungs.

twins, fraternal: Two embryos resulting from the fertilization of separate ova by separate sperm cells.

twins, identical: Two embryos resulting from the fertilization of a single egg cell by a single sperm that has separated into two separate parts.

typhoid fever: An intestinal infection caused by *Salmonella typhi*; also known as enteric fever.

U

ulcer (UL-ser): An open sore or erosion of the skin or mucous membrane resulting in tissue loss and usually with inflammation.

ulcer, decubitus: An ulcerated area caused by prolonged pressure that cuts off circulation to a body part; also known as a pressure ulcer or bedsore.

uremia (you-**REE**-mee-ah): A toxic condition caused by excessive amount of urea and other waste products in the bloodstream; also known as uremic poisoning.

ureterectasis (you-**ree**-ter-**ECK**-tah-sis): Distention of a ureter.

ureterolith (you-**REE**-ter-oh-**lith**): Presence of stones in a ureter.

ureterorrhagia (you-**ree**-ter-oh-**RAY**-jee-ah): Bleeding from the ureter.

ureterostenosis (you-**ree**-ter-oh-steh-**NOH**-sis): A stricture of the ureter.

urethralgia (**you**-ree-**THRAL**-jee-ah): Pain in the urethra.

urethritis (**you**-reh-**THRIGH**-tis): Inflammation of the urethra.

urethrocele (you-**REE**-throh-seel): Hernia in the urethral wall.

urethrorrhagia (you-**ree**-throh-**RAY**-jee-ah): Bleeding from the urethra.

urethrorrhea (you-**ree**-throh-**REE**-ah): An abnormal discharge from the urethra.

urethrostenosis (you-**ree**-throh-steh-**NOH**-sis): A stricture of the urethra.

urticaria (**ur**-tih-**KAR**-ree-ah): A skin condition characterized by localized areas of swelling accompanied by itching that is associated with an allergic reaction; also known as hives.

uveitis (**you**-vee-**EYE**-tis): Inflammation anywhere in the uveal tract.

V

vaginal candidiasis (**kan**-dih-**DYE**-ah-sis): A vaginal yeast infection caused by *Candida albicans*.

vaginitis (**vaj**-ih-**NIGH**-tis): Inflammation of the lining of the vagina; also known as colpitis.

vaginocele (**VAJ**-ih-noh-**seel**): Hernia protruding into the vagina; prolapse or falling down of the vagina.

vaginodynia (vaj-ih-noh-**DIN**-ee-ah): Pain in the vagina.

vaginosis, bacterial: A sexually transmitted bacterial infection of the vagina.

valvulitis (**val**-view-**LYE**-tis): Inflammation of a heart valve.

varicocele (**VAR**-ih-koh-**seel**): A varicose vein of the testicles that may cause male infertility.

varicose veins (**VAR**-ih-kohs **VAYNS**): Abnormally swollen veins.

vasculitis (**vas**-kyou-**LYE**-tis): Inflammation of a blood or lymph vessel; also known as angiitis.

venereal diseases (veh-**NEER**-ee-ahl): Diseases transmitted through sexual intercourse or other genital contact; also known as sexually transmitted diseases.

verrucae (veh-**ROO**-see): Skin lesions caused by the human papilloma virus; also known as warts.

vertigo (**VER**-tih-goh): A sense of whirling, dizziness, and the loss of balance.

vesicle (**VES**-ih-kul): A circumscribed elevation of skin containing fluid that is less than 0.5 cm in diameter; also known as a blister.

vesicovaginal fissure (**ves**-ih-koh-**VAJ**-ih-nahl): An abnormal opening between the bladder and vagina.

vitiligo (**vit**-ih-**LYE**-goh): A condition in which a loss of melanocytes results in whitish areas of skin bordered by normally pigmented areas.

volvulus (**VOL**-view-lus): Twisting of the intestine on itself that causes an obstruction.

vulvitis (vul-**VYE**-tis): Inflammation of the vulva.

vulvodynia (vul-voh-**DIN**-ee-ah): A nonspecific syndrome of unknown cause characterized by chronic burning, pain during sexual intercourse, itching, or stinging irritation of the vulva.

vulvovaginitis (**vul**-voh-**vaj**-ih-**NIGH**-tis): Inflammation of the vulva and the vagina.

X

xeroderma (zee-roh-**DER**-mah): Excessively dry skin.

xerophthalmia (**zeer**-ahf-**THAL**-mee-ah): Drying of eye surfaces characterized by the loss of luster of the conjunctiva and cornea.

Body Systems

■ ■ ■

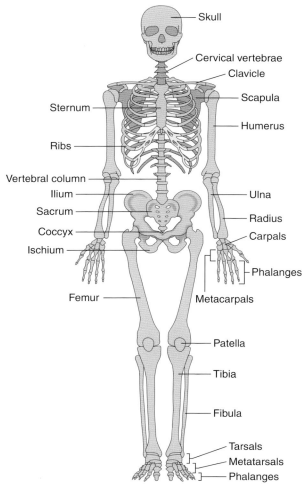

Anterior view of the adult human skeleton.

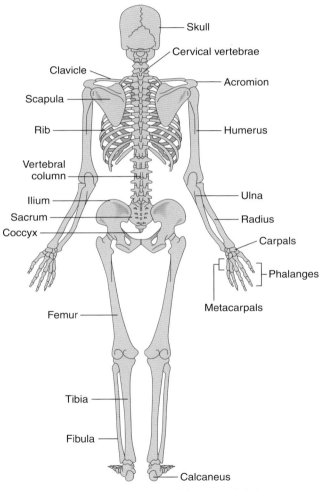

Posterior view of the adult human skeleton.

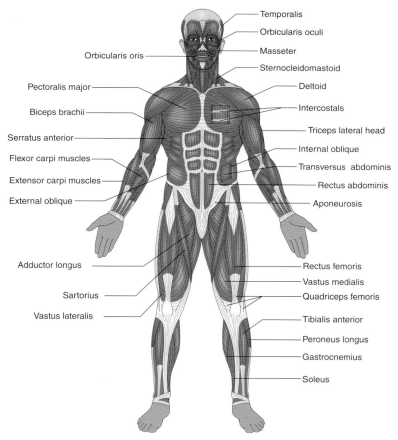

Temporalis
Orbicularis oculi
Orbicularis oris
Masseter
Sternocleidomastoid
Pectoralis major
Deltoid
Biceps brachii
Intercostals
Serratus anterior
Triceps lateral head
Flexor carpi muscles
Internal oblique
Extensor carpi muscles
Transversus abdominis
Rectus abdominis
External oblique
Aponeurosis
Adductor longus
Rectus femoris
Vastus medialis
Sartorius
Quadriceps femoris
Vastus lateralis
Tibialis anterior
Peroneus longus
Gastrocnemius
Soleus

Major muscles of body (anterior view).

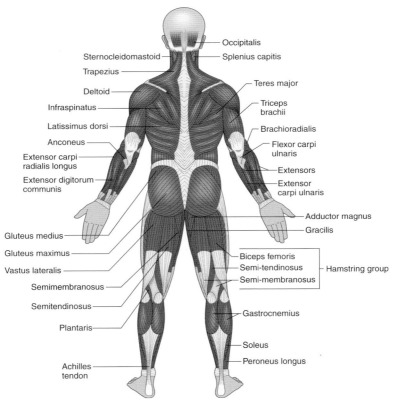

Major muscles of body (posterior view).

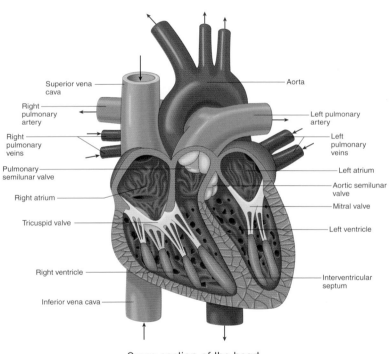

Superior vena cava

Right pulmonary artery

Right pulmonary veins

Pulmonary semilunar valve

Right atrium

Tricuspid valve

Right ventricle

Inferior vena cava

Aorta

Left pulmonary artery

Left pulmonary veins

Left atrium

Aortic semilunar valve

Mitral valve

Left ventricle

Interventricular septum

Cross section of the heart.

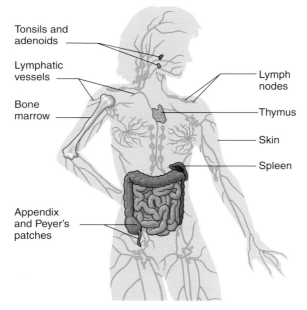

The immune system.

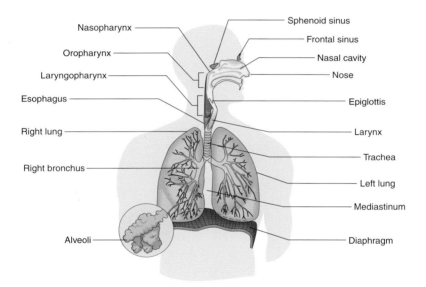

Respiratory system.

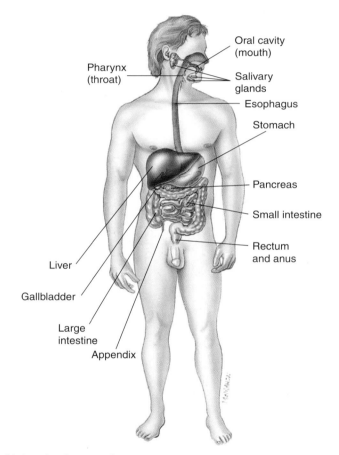

Major structures and accessory organs of the digestive system.

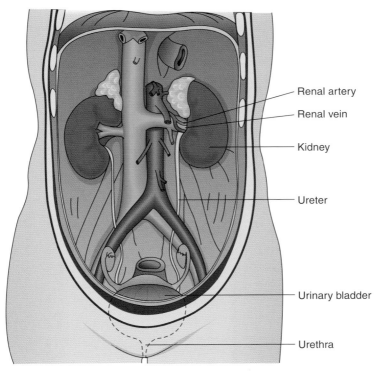

Renal artery

Renal vein

Kidney

Ureter

Urinary bladder

Urethra

Anterior view of the structures of the urinary system.

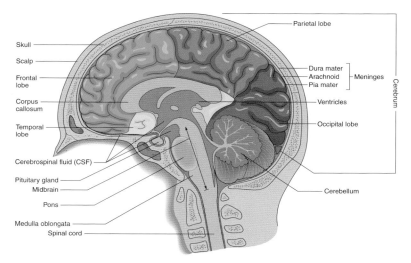

Cross section of the brain.

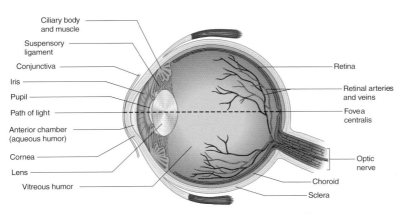

Ciliary body
and muscle

Suspensory
ligament

Conjunctiva

Iris

Pupil

Path of light

Anterior chamber
(aqueous humor)

Cornea

Lens

Vitreous humor

Retina

Retinal arteries
and veins

Fovea
centralis

Optic
nerve

Choroid

Sclera

Structures of the eyeball shown in cross section.

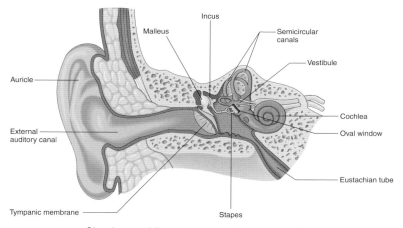

Structures of the ear shown in cross section.

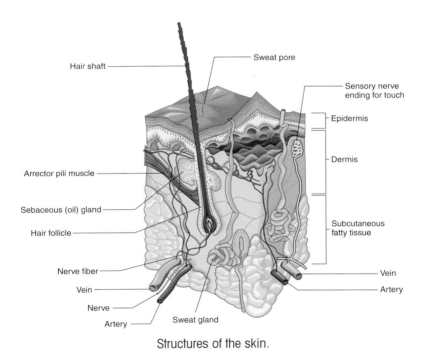

Hair shaft

Sweat pore

Sensory nerve
ending for touch

Epidermis

Dermis

Arrector pili muscle

Sebaceous (oil) gland

Hair follicle

Subcutaneous
fatty tissue

Nerve fiber

Vein

Vein

Nerve

Artery

Artery

Sweat gland

Structures of the skin.

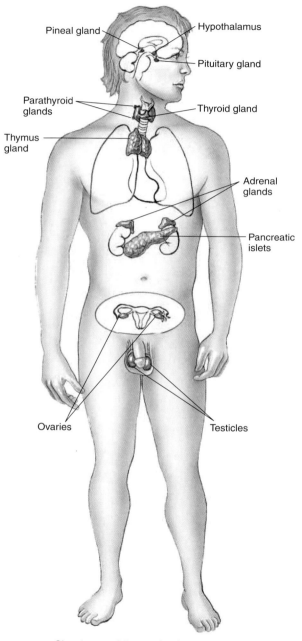

Structures of the endocrine system.

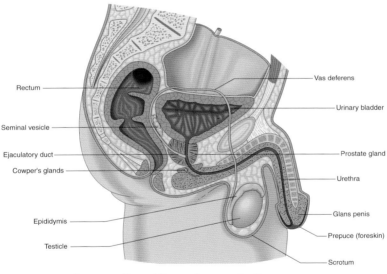

Cross section of the male reproductive organs.

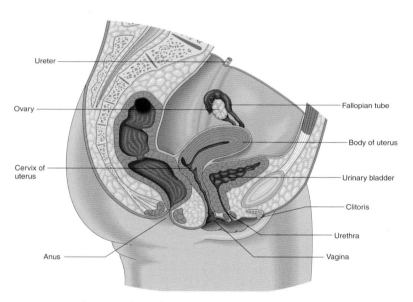

Cross section of the female reproductive organs.